"This guidebook serves as a very useful service delivery tool for SLPs and other related health care professionals. Stephanie LoPresti has used her background in psychology to develop the Protocol, focusing on a child development approach using the principles from developmental psychology. This work is highly appreciable."

Dr. Ramesh Bettagere, *PhD AuD CCC-SLP/A*

W0234984

The Speech and Language Protocol

This valuable book addresses the common problems faced by speech-language pathologists, offering solutions and strategies for more effective service delivery.

Stephanie LoPresti introduces 'The Protocol,' a child development-based approach that merges principles from developmental psychology and speech-language pathology. The book covers a wide range of speech and language issues, including receptive, expressive, pragmatic, feeding, and play development, making it a versatile resource for clinicians. It is designed to be easy to use, with movable elements that adapt to a child's progress from short- to long-term milestones and goals. It emphasizes the concept of the zone of proximal development, ensuring that clinicians work with clients just above their current level of functioning, leading to meaningful progress.

Accompanied by downloadable worksheets to assess progress, it will be an essential resource for all speech and language pathologists, particularly those working with young children. It will also be useful to students and educators in the field of speech-language pathology seeking evidence-based strategies for working with clients, as well as healthcare professionals, researchers, and educators interested in child development and language acquisition.

Stephanie LoPresti, MS CCC-SLP TSSLD, is a seasoned Certified Speech-Language Pathologist with a decade of diverse experience spanning medical and academic settings. With expertise in conducting comprehensive evaluations and implementing evidence-based interventions, she excels in managing caseloads, supervising clinical staff, and collaborating with multidisciplinary teams. Currently based in the United States, Stephanie's career has seen her impact the lives of clients from infancy to adulthood, specializing in areas such as autism spectrum disorders, dysphagia, and medically complex conditions across various regions including New York, Colorado, and California. For more personal details and to follow her journey, you can visit her website http://www.itsremotelyspeech.com and follow her on Instagram @itsremotelyspeech

The Speech and Language Protocol

An Assessment Tool for Early Years

Stephanie LoPresti

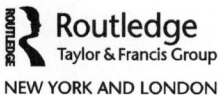

Routledge
Taylor & Francis Group

NEW YORK AND LONDON

Designed cover image: FluxFactory via Getty Images

First published 2025
by Routledge
605 Third Avenue, New York, NY 10158

and by Routledge
4 Park Square, Milton Park, Abingdon, Oxon, OX14 4RN

Routledge is an imprint of the Taylor & Francis Group, an informa business

© 2025 Stephanie LoPresti

Library of Congress Cataloging-in-Publication Data
Names: LoPresti, Stephanie, author.
Title: The speech and language protocol : an assessment tool for
early years / Stephanie LoPresti.
Description: New York, NY : Routledge, 2025. | Includes
bibliographical references and index. |
Identifiers: LCCN 2024028194 (print) | LCCN 2024028195
(ebook) | ISBN 9781032794136 (hbk) | ISBN 9781032742465
(pbk) | ISBN 9781003491842 (ebk)
Subjects: MESH: Speech-Language Pathology—methods | Language
Development | Language Disorders—diagnosis | Speech Disorders—
diagnosis | Child
Classification: LCC RC425 .L64 2025 (print) | LCC RC425
(ebook) | NLM WL 340.2 | DDC 616.85/5—dc23/eng/20240904
LC record available at https://lccn.loc.gov/2024028194
LC ebook record available at https://lccn.loc.gov/2024028195

ISBN: 978-1-032-79413-6 (hbk)
ISBN: 978-1-032-74246-5 (pbk)
ISBN: 978-1-003-49184-2 (ebk)

DOI: 10.4324/9781003491842

Typeset in Sabon
by codeMantra

Access the Support Material: www.routledge.com/9781032742465

Contents

1 Introduction

After working over ten years in our wonderful and, at times, all-encompassing career of speech-language pathology, there was a common theme or problem (rather) that I noticed which followed me throughout my differing settings in which I provided service to my clients.

That problem was a lack in organization with testing and its bridge between an assessment and service delivery or therapy. A particular area of weakness was in the preschool population where I often found myself spending hours doing one of the two things: (1) looking for up-to-date developmental milestones and (2) finding an assessment that 'had it all'; an assessment where I can provide families what is 'average/expected development,' how their child is functioning in relation to that, and (this last part is what makes The Protocol different) the targets between where they are and where they are going in order to create a clear and succinct roadmap between where they are and the road they have to take to succeed.

The Protocol marks the child's highest ability in a particular area (e.g. social milestones), compares it to norms with children their age, and will mark the next sequential step (e.g. their 'zone of proximal development') (Mcleod, 2024), where therapy goals can easily be attained and carried over at home. Incremental steps that are *just* hard enough, with guided interventionists, can be successfully targeted to reach those age-appropriate milestones.

There are three things we need to know in order to make progress in any area: where the child is functioning currently, where we are going, and the steps that are needed to attain the end goal. Through this evaluation and service delivery method, the track to success will be clear to speech-language pathologists, their clients, and the families they serve. We do not have the time to be searching for methods which will yield success on a daily basis; this is the problem that The Protocol solves. It takes the 'guesswork' out of assessment, daily treatment, and impromptu meetings with families and educators. The Protocol is a true roadmap to success for speech-language pathologists.

DOI: 10.4324/9781003491842-1

Core Principles of the Protocol

This is to be used as a guidepost to effective service delivery with the vision to always be working on specific incremental goals that are just above the client's current level of functioning in order to yield real results.

We are talking about the well-known and researched concept published by Vygotsky in 1962, the zone of proximal development. With The Protocol, you will be using the zone of proximal development with successive approximation by taking the client's current level of functioning and working ONE developmental step above where they are functioning. These small and incremental milestones are just hard enough where they are learning a new skill, BUT that they can successfully learn with your clinical intervention as a speech-language pathologist.

I have developed the protocol for the following core reason: I believe in the research behind typical developmental milestones and how the brain wires itself based on years of research. However, there has yet to be a method in which to harness this invaluable information into a clear, concise, and functional method to inspire success with our clients meeting and exceeding those milestones. By completing The Protocol with your clients, my vision is to make everyday therapy easier to track progress, meet your clients where they are, set them up for success (since you will be working in their zone of proximal development, which is always moving as they are progressing in their explicit speech instruction), and inspire meaningful change in their lives.

Let this protocol take the guesswork out of your client's weekly targets in therapy and work WITH their brains natural course of development.

How to Utilize The Protocol

The workbook at the end of this text will be located and referenced in the appendix for ease in utilization of The Protocol. In addition, an online 'Protocol Calculator' can be utilized which determines the 'zone of intervention' for your use.

Steps to quick determination of the child's zone of intervention:

Highlight the stage they have mastered completely (their level of mastery) and identify the stage just above (more advanced) than their current level of functioning. This is the child's zone of intervention.

Use this stage to generate short-term session goals in order to assist in mastery of this next stage through repetition and language expansion strategies.

I have added age expectations in your graph as this is the 'end goal' of our therapy, but it also serves as a guide when explaining the level of weakness.

Personal Background

I believe the idea for The Protocol has not been an overnight epiphany, so to say, but rather, a culmination of experiences and areas of potential development to explore in the field. To provide a bit of personal context to this work, I would love to share accounts which have driven my interest in developing this tool for my fellow speech-pathologists.

For context, I will bring personal accounts in the form of case studies that pertain to the differing areas in which I explore in The Protocol. The personal accounts come from the settings in which I have worked as a speech- language pathologist.

I set out on my path to become a speech-language pathologist later than some. Being a child of a special education teacher and public school administrator, some would say that this profession was "in my bones." Many of my family members have been in the 'helping' professions in one way or another; whether it be a general medical practitioner, a nurse, a psychologist, or in some realm of education, I have always sought out to help others through my work. With my family background in mind, I decided to major in psychology for my undergraduate degree. The most interesting portion of psychology for me, personally, revolved around child development. I was particularly fascinated by the theories that explain how and why children develop in typical or atypical ways. This is when I was introduced to the lovely field of speech-language pathology in an extended school year position as a personal aide for a young child with Rett's disorder. I will share more on this particular experience later, however; this marked a particularly significant calling to the field of an SLP (speech-language pathologist). Being a semi 'typical' undergraduate, this meant I needed to acquire the pre-requisite courses that would enable me to apply for graduate school. During this time, I had worked part time in a private pediatric therapy center, shadowing speech, occupational, and physical therapists as well as submitting insurance billing for reimbursement for the company. Having completed my prerequisite courses for admission mid-year led me to the graduate school I attended and acquired my graduate degree, Southeastern Louisiana University. So, a girl from the northeast relocated to Hammond, Louisiana, a mere 45 minutes from New Orleans, the location of all my clinical externships.

I can remember, as if it were yesterday, learning about the vast depth of areas in the field of speech-language pathology. Therefore, I sought out work across various settings in order to add enrichment to my personal clinical experience. While I began my rotation in an elementary school, my sequential experiences were in the medical sector of the profession. While these areas of the field may be seen in complete opposition, there have been varying similarities up to and including the fact that psychology and basic counseling principles I learned in undergraduate greatly assisted me in service delivery across all settings and all ages.

My first pediatric medical setting was at Children's Hospital of New Orleans, where I completed a clinical rotation at an outpatient office of the main campus. Children who visited my supervisor (let's call her Megan) and myself ranged from the increasingly medically complex including children with severe apraxia of speech, to cerebral palsy, to children with multiple medical disabilities. I can still picture the first experience I had with a child who had not only childhood apraxia of speech but also an apraxic gait. For those of you who want a quick update on this verbiage, gait is the manner of walking or moving across a room. This was visibly quite distinct, as he would be found literally running into a table that is in the corner of the room, his gait was rather staggered and not unlike an adult who was, for lack of a better word, inebriated. I learned to quickly tailor the method of intervention for each child. As intervention with a child with apraxia varies greatly from other interventions utilized for a child with receptive language deficits or a cerebral palsy. If I had to pinpoint the interest in milestones as they relate to the field of speech-language pathology, I would have to say that this particular experience in Children's Hospital of New Orleans planted the seed for my Protocol project. In particular, I recall googling 'cognitive milestone expectations' from the Dell computer in my supervisor's room in order to provide a basis on which to effectively meet my young client's where they were currently functioning.

From Children's Hospital of New Orleans, I took my last internship at Touro Neurological Rehabilitation Hospital in the beautiful garden district of New Orleans. I was particularly interested in this placement as, word on the street, my 'to-be' supervisor was "as tough as they came" and an excellent teacher. This experience, under the supervision of "Miss Rynn," marked my first experience working with adults who spanned from the inpatient intensive care with patients who were in a coma state to a 36-year-old law school graduate who fell from a second-story balcony during a night of celebration who consequently had a severe traumatic brain injury as a result. One of the last clients I had while working under Miss Rynn's supervision was a 31-year-old audiologist who was found on the floor by her husband, having had a cerebrovascular attack (CVA) while she was in labor with her child. You may be thinking at this point, where does The Protocol come into development in such a setting? For my speech-pathologist colleagues who have worked with adults, there are various parallels between language and speech acquisition and later speech RE-acquisition after neurological events. While The Protocol you will read is geared toward younger children, I input my experience with adults as I have utilized the same methods with my adult patients as it relates to successive steps toward a return to their 'baseline.' Baseline is their prior level of performance before the incident, event, or gradual decline if we are addressing a progressive disease (e.g. Alzheimer's dementia, Amyotrophic Lateral Sclerosis, or Parkinson's disease).

Following my graduation from Southeastern Louisiana University, I took a job in Boulder County of Colorado working in one of their international elementary schools and further headstart programs for preschoolers. For those of you who are not familiar with the United States Head Start program, it is a "program run by the United States Department of Health and Human Services that provides comprehensive early childhood education, health, nutrition and parent involvement services to low-income children and families" (*Head start services*, 2023). I can still remember the first day working as a speech-pathologist, listening to the children rehearsing for a play of which I could hear from my small office that overlooked the beautiful foothills of Boulder county's mountains. What stood out in this particular position was my exposure to children who were international in their backgrounds. I was blessed to work closely with children of various ethnic backgrounds whose parents spoke both English and many of which required translation. The Head Start children I serviced could also have attributed to my interest in 'typical child development.' I spent many hours rifling through old treatment textbooks in order to put together my own 'screeners' whenever I received a Head Start referral for potential speech and language services. In fact, as I write about this experience, I recall that I utilized these screeners to format my written assessments as many of the younger population can be rather 'untestable' by standardized testing protocol standards. I still recall my sense of pride with the completion of these reports, as I was able to provide teachers, aides, and family members with invaluable information on where their child lies in relation to their same-age peers.

From my work in Colorado, I finished up my clinical fellowship year in subacute and long-term care facilities, first in Houston, Texas, and last on the shore of New Jersey. This shift was rather intentional, as I sought to be "competent" in any setting that I was placed in, and this setting was one in which I had, admittedly, no experience prior to the second half of my clinical fellowship (CF) year. To provide context, a clinical fellowship year in the United States is the first 36 weeks in which a speech-pathologist graduate is working under the supervision or mentorship of a more seasoned speech-pathologist. The idea is that you will gain access to another speech-language pathologist to ask questions and to review your documentation as well as clinical service delivery. While my first experience working in the SNF (skilled nursing facility) was under supervision, I do feel that I learned the documentation and methods by shadowing the speech-pathologist I was taking over for. As you may imagine, much of my caseload encompassed working on dysphagia, dementia, dysarthria, and even some CVA (cerebrovascular accidents) cases which yielded residual anomia and word-finding deficits. You may be thinking to yourself, how does The Protocol tie in here, as it is an entirely different part of life or scope rather? Intervention with the adult population again was based on functionality of both communication and swallowing (aka dysphagia). I was able to see the vast connection between dysphagia (swallowing) and meal consumption to social communication and connection. This clinical experience really solidified and set me up for success in my later work with pediatric dysphagia and feeding cases in which I served children in New York City's early intervention program. My work with the adults drew heavily on my psychology background, as not only do they need to be convinced that you are assisting them in a 'respectful' way, but rather that you can counsel and educate the families in the process to achieve real progress. Further on in my introduction, I will touch on the topic of 'point of interest' which has vastly impacted my service delivery to patients across the age span. This is evident in my adult population (as well as my pediatric population), as you can gain trust and develop real working relationships with clients. This is accomplished by discovering where they come from and what they did for a living, by acknowledging and really seeing what 'makes them tick.' As far as reference to the development of The Protocol while I have worked with the adult population, I have utilized successive approximation and progression from what an adult is currently able to swallow, advancing them to the least restrictive diet. This has also been evident with the motor speech progressions portion of The Protocol, as well as from a language perspective, to assist with word finding and anomia which is comorbid with clients who have aphasia.

From my work with adults in the skilled nursing facility, I was drawn back to working with my pediatric population. I had experienced my first position working with multi-disabilities children deep in Brooklyn where augmentative and alternative communication (AAC devices) and picture exchange communication systems (PECS) were being used. These children ranged from 8 years to 21 years of age (Bondy, 2023). This particular population was more of a clear representation of what I will reference later when we speak about Brown's Stages and further cognitive milestones, in which some children simply do not attain the later acquisitioning abilities. The scope and depth of practice and intervention with the children in this position were based on functionality of skills. I enjoyed assisting in offering the children their voice by teaching functional communication measures through the utilization of a very basic augmentative and alternative communication (AAC) device with associated contingencies. In thinking back on this experience, I learned the benefit of utilization of binary choice. Binary choice is basically the choice between two; while a child has a higher percentage of accuracy (50%), I would shift the location and position of objects in my hands while providing this choice to identify if they were preferring one side or actually scanning the objects I was directing them to select. The population which is more cognitively impaired improved their functional communication skills vastly through a multi-modal approach to teaching skills. I learned the true value of going through the steps required to assist in attainment of a new skill. What does this look like? More discrete trials of "I push a button, I get the veggie stick" and various cause and effect of behavior. This particular setting was one in which I was able to work alongside Applied Behavioral Analysts (ABA) professionals, to glean the insights behind their training in a behavioral approach to teaching imperative skills. I will link information on Applied Behavioral Analysis below, as I do believe there is value in their work, and they have proven to be an important resource to me throughout my work as a speech-language pathologist across differing settings. While I was able to glean a depth of insights into this particular population, I felt the drive to return to the younger population, which led me to my next position in the field.

I had spent the better part of five years working in the Upper West Side of Manhattan at an organization which used to be known as United Cerebral Palsy (or UCP) and has since shifted to Adapt Community Network. In this particular position, I worked with children of varying abilities and disabilities in one of New York City's private preschools. This is when I 'took on' the job of working as the speech departments 'craft' consultant. I worked tirelessly to put together themed activities that coordinated with thematic and age-appropriate books for the children we served in the speech room. I had rather loved this position as I was able to use my creativity to develop a kind of curriculum for the children we served, utilizing the standard goals to enrich our child's learning with 'hands on' play and exploration. Direction following and prepositional phrases are riddled throughout the completion of a craft or activity. Besides my hobby of speech curriculum development in that position, I began seeing particular areas of need as it related to tracking of service delivery and even assessment with the younger population. The standard batteries that we utilized included Preschool Language Scale and Goldman Fristoe Test of Articulation to assess where a child needed intervention. However, for my seasoned speech-pathologists, we know that a large group of our clients are 'formally untestable,' and the standard score of 50 and below did not provide insight for educators, parents, or ourselves on 'steps to take' or a baseline of speech and language functioning. I recall complaining, probably ad nauseam to my colleagues, about the time spent to ascertain a score or rather functional measure of exactly where our children were in their speech and language development and a need for a tool to succinctly calculate this for us to lead to effective service delivery.

At the same time that I was working at United Cerebral Palsy, I was introduced to the early intervention of the field. For those of you who are unfamiliar with this term, the New York State Early Intervention Program (EIP) is part of the national Early Intervention Program for infants and toddlers with disabilities and their families. To be eligible for services, "children must be under 3 years of age and have a confirmed disability or established developmental delay, as defined by the State, in one or more of the following areas of development: physical, cognitive, communication, social-emotional and/or adaptive" (*Department of Health: Early Intervention Program*, 1993). What makes the early intervention setting so unique is that all services are carried out in the clients home (or daycare) where skills can be taught IN the actual context of daily life. This setting provides the intersection between providers and parents who are with their children a majority of the day. Over my years working in the early intervention sector (EI), I developed a sort of 'elevator pitch' to parents: "While I am with your child, on average of 60 minutes a week, you are with them the rest of the 95% of the time; so any progress that is made is made from OUR work together." This catch phrase not only helped with family buy-in, but also with ongoing parental training or coaching approach to language and feeding acquisition skills and methods. In reflecting back over my professional life when I worked as an early interventionist, I recall this time as being a 'hustle' as most of the time (after my full-time job) I could be spotted on the one, two, or three NYC subways with an extra-large Heschl backpack that held all of my speech toys in their individual 'plastic baggies' as communicative ploys for the little ones. I still provide early intervention to spare families in the community to keep my 'hands,' so-to-say, in this vital area of the field. The children I came across in this area of the field varied, as well, all the way from a baby who was diagnosed with Moebius syndrome at birth and needed feeding and communication intervention, to children on the autism spectrum, to multiples who were pure "later language acquisitioning." Early intervention was an area, in particular, where I was riddled with questions related to 'age expectations and milestones' across disciplines. Such questions like "when can I expect my baby to eat solid foods, how much should my child be saying, should he be following directions at this age?, etc.," really led to my avid online searching related to milestones and expectations to share with the families I had grown so close to. While this area of the field has yielded the most improvement amongst the clients and families I served, there was always a relative sadness related to diagnoses that were realized or shared with families around this time. Often early interventionists are more of the 'frontline workers' who can first identify areas of deficits that can indicate a greater developmental disability which can greatly impact these families in the long run. What I had and have provided families whose children are in this age range is the knowledge and milestones associated with a child of the same age as their own babies. With this information, they can make informed decisions on the treatment and path of their little ones moving forward.

From my time working at United Cerebral Palsy, I had acquired a position in New York City Public Schools. In this position, I worked in both a specialized music school, where a large number of the caseload encompassed children who were functioning higher on-the-autism spectrum and some attention deficit disorders which required executive functioning training (e.g. organizational and scheduling skills), with a vast emphasis on metalinguistic skills. Metalinguistic skills being those higher level language skills that are often associated with pragmatic deficits (e.g. reading body language, inferencing, social cues). This particular setting is where I developed the belief that we are all given certain strengths and weaknesses when we are born, and we can often use those strengths to offset the weaknesses. This, in particular, is another area where the concept of 'getting on their level' is crucial, as children who have such a vast ability in certain areas (like these children's musical abilities) may have differing priorities and interests than the layman elementary schooler. In the specialized music school, I often referred to pragmatic milestones, as they even related back to as basic as the concept of theory of mind. Theory of mind refers to "the ability to attribute mental states to oneself and others" which can include "understanding that other people's beliefs, desires, intentions, emotions and thoughts may differ from their own." As suggested by researchers, theory of mind (ToM) serves as "foundational elements for social interaction" (Ruhl, 2023).

Another school in which I had worked in New York City: Department of Education was a bilingual middle school, particularly one of which was half French speaking. My caseload in this school ranged from children who had generalized learning disabilities such as attention deficit disorder (ADD) and attention deficit hyperactivity disorder (ADHD), to children who had specific language impairments as they related to expressive and, in particular, written language. I additionally had one child who had dysarthric speech secondary to his traumatic birth, of which we targeted the rate and coarticulation of his speech but in the context of academic work he was completing. I can still remember "Johnny" let's call him showing me a newspaper clipping of "this Chinese government built hospitals to house patients who had this mysterious illness known as COVID-19" needless to say, there were a number of instances where Johnny brought to light wisdom and information that made him seem as he was wise well beyond his years. I will mention my time working with "my middle schoolers" as I coined them frequently in the upcoming pages of The Protocol, as many of the milestones and utilization of core learning strategies (e.g. scaffolding, modeling, recasting, preparatory sets) greatly impacted my students and their receptive and expressive language development. In correlating with grammatical rules, in particular, with written language, I often pulled out Brown's stages of development (to be referenced in depth later on) to assist in their 'correction' of their own texts. While 'written language' was a real SELL to middle schoolers who resided in the Upper West Side of Manhattan, I would often find opportunities to drop pitches for the 'cause' as they were expressing their middle school 'gripes' of the day as they entered the speech room. I could be heard saying something along the lines of "You have a lot to say. Does it feel like they are not listening? You know another way you can tell them your problem"... "let's write it down for them." I would let them know that THEIR voice is important, to not silence themselves because they "don't have time" to write down their thoughts. This was particularly effective when it came to social issues and persuasion pieces, of which were an all-time interest to my middle schoolers.

I worked in New York City Public Schools before and during the COVID-19 pandemic, even when we transitioned to entirely remote learning. I found it fascinating how my tech-savvy middle schoolers were able to utilize calendar apps and the computer to actually be texting ME about their upcoming 'speech class.' If nothing else, their executive functioning skills benefited from the organization of a virtual calendar with embedded reminders. As a reminder, "executive function" describes a set of cognitive processes and mental skills that help an individual plan, monitor, and successfully execute their goals. The 'executive functions,' as they're known, include "attentional control, working memory, inhibition and problem solving" (*Executive function*, 2020). Either way, I was able to quickly pivot from in-person intervention to entirely remote intervention with not only my middle schoolers, but ALSO my early intervention families. The 'heavy lifting' as we could call it of being in person with the early intervention babies was completed directly by their family members, all the time. This meant that if the parents were "all hands on deck" with intervention, their children would be getting 'therapy' through their parents carrying over the skills taught to them by myself, and other therapists.

Following the "return to normal" as we called it in the United States, I decided to take on travel therapy positions in other cities in the United States. The first of which was in Denver, Colorado Public Schools. I was in a nice area of the city where the parents advocated having their children in school from 8 to 4 or 5:00 pm. Here, I conducted therapy and caseload management for an excess of 80 children ages from preschool inclusion classrooms through the eighth grade. Of course, the preschool classrooms remained my favored crowd, as I was able to collaborate closely with the special education teachers as well as provide support to the parents and educators as they relate to typical child development. My caseload in

Denver spanned from children who were primarily non-verbal and on the autism spectrum, to children who had pervasive phonological disorders (I had an innumerable amount of second graders who fronted their backed sounds), to children who were in middle school and were exhibiting stuttering like characteristics and were eventually classified. Again, with the increase in caseload, I felt the need for succinct data collection and personal check-ins with the child's current level of functioning to determine daily and weekly treatment targets. At this juncture, I was utilizing The Protocol, updating milestones as they were researched, for my own purposes of service delivery. In particular, due to the vast majority of students who were being treated for articulation disorders, I would utilize norm-referenced milestones as a method to target successive speech sound errors as they progressed for level of complexity. Another point I would like to add here is my improved professional skill of conducting a stuttering assessment, both formally and informally and the further knowledge I had begun to share with families and teachers of discrepancies between "normal developmental nonfluencies" and a "true stutter." I would review 'normal developmental nonfluencies' and their association with stress and pressure as well as the distinction between this and a true stutter or abnormality. While The Protocol does not have a section on dysfluencies and stuttering, I utilized the same concepts of sequential steps as they relate to increasing utterance length (and sentence complexity) while diminishing dysfluencies.

After my time in Denver, I accepted a travel position in Boston Public Schools, where I was covering maternity leave in a multi-disability school which ranged from preschool through eighth grade. The school had inclusion with applied behavioral analysts (ABA) and therefore, I was working alongside various ABA therapists during sessions both inside and outside of the classroom. Nearly half of the population which I had seen in the school were either on the autism spectrum or had various cognitive disabilities, leaving the collaboration with ABA and my background knowledge in behavioral principles paramount to effective service delivery. There was a clear distinction between the children who had received ABA 'earlier' in their academic career, such as the preschoolers, and those later on, such as middle schoolers. This time is one spent on very small 'incremental' targets to improve a child's functional communication.

From the maternity coverage, I took a position working in a skilled nursing facility (SNF) with a large subacute section in South Boston where I remained until I moved back to the greater New York area. This year was one in which I spent innumerable hours of overtime (as I was covering for the director who was on maternity leave) with the patients in the subacute section of the facility. In this particular setting, I drew on my psychology background to establish and improve rapport with the clients and their families, thus, improving therapy buy in. Many of my patients had experienced cerebrovascular attacks (CVA's), throat and neck cancer, sudden falls and broken hips, Parkinson's, as well as advancing Alzheimer's dementia. Again, I targeted the successive approximation approach to 'baby steps' more closely approximating my patient's 'baseline.' For some, admittedly, I served as an advocate for improved quality of life. I still remember a patient who had end-stage throat cancer; when I went into the room for a bedside swallow evaluation he whispered in my direction if I could bring him something comforting, "Do you have an ice pop?" Needless to say, I ensured the last seven days he was with us in this life that every nurse knew the ice pops in the freezer were to be offered to him whenever they entered that room. Many of the further interventions I utilized with patients who exhibited a version of anomia (loss of word finding) secondary to cognitive overload or potential development of dementia were not unlike the interventions I utilized with middle schoolers. Various learning strategies such as scaffolding, fill in the blank, and phonetic cues were invaluable in assisting in the rewiring of the neuronal pathways of the brain.

Eventually, I made my way back to the greater New York City area, where I presently reside. My current work encompasses working part-time position in UPK (universal preschool) for children who have disabilities, and online caseload management and SLPA (speech-language pathology assistants) remotely, part time. My current days are jam packed between direct intervention in the preschool sector, at a little school in the Throggs Neck location of the Bronx; accompanied by days in which I fill either directly supervising SLPAs virtually and/or conducting online assessments and IEP meetings with school-aged children from preschool through 18 years. Many of my case studies will additionally be drawn from my current work with the diverse pediatric population I serve both in the academic and pre-academic sectors. Needless to say, the publishing of The Protocol has really come at a personally important time of my life, as I feel the need to utilize and share such a tool to assist in effective service delivery and assessment of the vast population in which I serve. If you have made it through my biography or chronology of events in my speech-pathology life, welcome and thank you for listening to the 'context' behind the stories and preceding to the development of The Protocol.

References

The Administration for Children and Families. (2023). *Head start services*. https://www.acf.hhs.gov/ohs/about/head-start

Bondy, A. (2023, April 17). *PECS®: An evidence-based practice*. Pyramid Educational Consultants. https://pecsusa.com/pecs/

New York State Department of Health. (1993). *Department of Health: Early Intervention Program.* https://www.health.ny.gov/community/infants_children/early_intervention/

Ruhl, C. (2023, August 28). What is theory of mind in psychology? *Simply Psychology.* https://www.simplypsychology.org/theory-of-mind.html

Sussex Publishers. (2020). Executive function. *Psychology Today.* https://www.psychologytoday.com/us/basics/executive-function

2   Foundational Information

Overview and Child Psychology Basis

The basis for development of the speech and language protocol rewinds back to studies in psychology. Having an undergraduate degree in psychology, many of the core concepts that intrigued me were based on development as well as normal and abnormal behaviors. A basic knowledge of psychology and its principles permits me to not only empathize with and understand my clients but also their family members. From a larger perspective, it can assist in gaining insight regarding both behavior, cognition, and learning, in general. I will reference my time working in the early intervention sector, where I cannot count the number of times that parents have approached me with questions such as "What SHOULD my child do at this age?" and "How should they sound?" I have always found this inquiry personally interesting and would base my answers after I have conducted personal research in order to guide them appropriately. ·

After a parent realizes their child is below or well below average in certain areas, the question is usually "What can I do?" or even "Is there any way my child can catch up with his peers?" This is when I explain how speech and language therapy assists in bridging the gap between where a child is currently functioning and where they *should* be functioning. This, I believe, is our gift that we give to the clients and families we work with.

When I speak about bridging that gap and providing a child with just enough interventions and methods to lead them to that next step, I realize I am describing a very distinct method as named and outlined by the famous psychologist Lev Vyzotsky, which is the "zone of proximal development." The zone of proximal development is the gap between what a child is doing independently and what they can do with the help of others (e.g. speech-language pathologists). Why is this important, according to the famous cognitive psychologist? Within the zone of proximal development, tasks that are just higher than a child's current abilities is the area

DOI: 10.4324/9781003491842-2

where instruction is most beneficial (and are even researched) to promote cognitive growth.

This is where it hit me. We (meaning speech-pathologists and any skilled interventionist) serve as guides to take our children from where they are to where they are meant to be. In Vygotsky's terms, the methods that we utilize can qualify us as filling the role of our children's "more knowledge-able other" (MKO). What is the role of a "more knowledgeable other"? This is someone who has a higher level of understanding or mastery than the learner in certain areas. While more knowledgeable others (MKO) can be peers (cue, social learning theory (Mcleod, 2024)), older brothers and sisters, parents, teachers, etc., Speech-language pathologists can step into the MKO role for the children and families we serve.

However, a common problem that I see almost in every report that I have read is the discrepancy between the test scores and where the child is currently functioning. Meaning, I can read innumerable amounts of initial evaluations and still have no clue what is walking in the door for the first session with my clients. I may have a vague idea of what the child can do, but as we know, no two children present the same, and it is imperative for clinicians to see exactly where and how they are functioning to make any type of progress. Who wants to grasp at straws during a session? This is the real everyday problem that The Protocol is aiming to solve.

Social learning theory was developed by a psychologist named Albert Bandura. According to Bandura's social learning theory (or SLT), "people learn new behaviors by observing and imitating others" (McLeod, 2020). Basically, through observational learning our children can acquire various skills, knowledge, and beliefs by watching the actions of others and the consequences that follow those behaviors. It is truly the correlation between both environmental and cognitive factors that merge together to influence both learning and behavior. Without completing a deep dive into social learning theory here, I have often referenced social learning theory daily. A personal example occurred just this morning while I was grabbing coffee with my 4-year-old Rhodesian Ridgeback, a 5-year-old boy saw her and made a comment to his mother. This interaction led to her son's affinity for dogs and later to her personal dismay to have to drop him at 'daycare' this morning. I had mentioned the importance of social learning theory from his peers in such a setting even at the cost of her one-on-one time with her son. The child's attendance at preschool is vital, as he will learn many skills through social learning theory and the models his peers will provide to him that his mother cannot teach him at home. As you can see, psychological theories hold true and can often guide our decisions related to childcare.

Answering the 'Why behind Intervention'

As I'm sure you are aware, there is actually a stage of development where we expect children to ask 'why' questions, between 2 and 5 years of age. The asking of 'why' demonstrates a further inquiry behind rationalization and reasoning. I like to refer to it as 'the method behind my madness' when I started working in the home early intervention setting, over 6 years ago. I think that this answering of a question (that wasn't always verbally asked) stemmed back to my time interning in a first-class trauma hospital down in New Orleans, Louisiana. I had received the rotation after much push on my end, after hearing that this externship was 'the best.' I still remember my first day in the rehabilitation office while my supervisor, Miss Rynn (name changed for privacy purposes), and I were pouring over patient files for the upcoming day. She programmed two questions into my subconscious at that time, one of which I have since negated but the other of which has stuck with me. The queries were: (1) upon reading a patient's file you should be able to know what they expect while they are walking in the door (e.g. left paralysis, slurred speech, etc.); and (2) you need to be able to answer the 'why' behind every intervention you provide to a patient. You may be thinking, let's pause – did she actually say this and, second, did she follow through? The answer to both questions was a resounding "yes." She would ask me the rationale behind *every* intervention I performed on patients who attended speech sessions in the hospital. And I would like to thank her for this, over ten years later. I feel that knowing the 'why' has served not only me but every single patient (or child) who has walked in my door for intervention.

What is the reason for asking ourselves the 'why' before performing any intervention? It allows us to critically think about three important variables: (1) Where a child is currently functioning, (2) where they are going, and (3) the intervention we provide will help them get from where they are functioning to where they are going. Therefore, I expect parents to ask the 'why' behind the reason I have a million clear plastic bags with toys in them, why I keep my toys in a bag and wait for the child to functionally request I take them out, the method behind my 'reading' a book without even uttering a word from the pages. I think that this connection helps not only with 'buy-in' from caregivers and colleagues, but it helps my mental reconstruction of what step I am guiding my client along their path to success.

While I have spent much of my time as a speech-language pathologist running back to the checklists and showing a parent where their child is and what subsequent skill I was working on I thought, there must be an easier way! This is where I have adapted The Protocol, with a sample below, of the information I provide to parents from the first private session I conduct with their child. I typically provide a 'range' of acquired skills in which we would be working toward in our weekly sessions. This information provided to parents from 'day one' has assisted in answering their questions about their child's current functioning in relation to their peers.

I am a visual person, so anything that is written out or drawn out for me is easier for me to comprehend. In fact, so much so that I would spend hours during comprehensive examinations drawing out cranial nerves, making posters with color-coded facts on the differing areas of deficits, etc. With a comprehensive visual, I have found my daily interventions easier to support and share with teachers and parents alike. I think in the process of sharing this method, I have even gotten some teachers excited about the concepts and development as a whole. Refer to the bottom of this section for a 'sample' visual for parents and teachers to assist with identifying the milestones for a particular age range.

I believe the most clear example of knowing the 'why' behind specific interventions can be demonstrated with a personal story of which I believe many other speech-language pathologists can empathize with. You know the student, the 2- or 3-year-old who could sit in a corner playing with a balloon for, literally, hours. Mine is a student who just so happens to love plastic bags. She loves pulling them from every cubby she can find, every trash can, and every glove box. Plastic bags and popping them were Mandy's favorite things in life. So much so that the classroom was inundated with playing a game of 'keep away' with Mandy to avoid her 'dumpster diving' for the entirety of the school day. Knowing that Mandy also had a proclivity for biting when she got angry, I knew that establishing rapport and getting ON Mandy's level would be crucial for development of a good working relationship with her. So, what did I do during the first two weeks of therapy with Mandy? We went down to the 'snoozlin' room with all the bouncy devices AND padded walls and would jump and end the session with her beloved bags. To an outsider, or untrained eye, this may look like merely 'passing the time' as we were both jumping and I was directly imitating her vocalizations and actions. However, about a week in not only did Mandy greet me FUNCTIONALLY at the door, by running up and hugging while approximating a sing-songy 'hi!' but she further established joint attention with me with shared eye contact and even during one session stopped her jumping to push my legs down into the chair – so I wouldn't be jumping around the classroom. Slowly Mandy was able to meet astronomical goals all because I knew the 'why' behind the interventions I was utilizing in our daily sessions. If anyone were to want to 'listen' to my explanation of the 'why,' I would be able to pull out the subsequent developmental milestones that we were sitting in during our wild 'workout' sessions that we had together. Needless to say, I know the why, and the why eventually became the 'how' of Mandy reaching some pivotal milestones.

Sample Informational Sheet for Parents/Educators, the below information comes from The Protocol, which is placed, in its entirety at the end of the book:

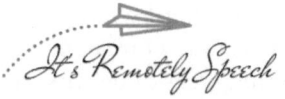

I break down speech/language, social, and preacademic milestones into subsequent charts for your review! These guide my recommendations (re: the appropriateness of therapy as well as goals for each client).

3–4-year-old milestones:

Play Expectations:

Parallel play (2.5–3.5 years)	Play is still solo but often alongside/next to other children
Associative play (3–4.5 years)	Begin to play with others by sharing toys

Academic-based milestones (from 30 months to 4 years):

Begins pretend play (e.g. feeding baby doll)
Demonstrates simple problem-solving skills (e.g. stands on stool to reach counter)
Follows two-step directions (e.g. get your shoes and bring them to the door)
Knows at least one color (e.g. show me blue)
Can draw a circle with direct model
Avoids touching hot stove when given warning (safety awareness)
Can label a number of colors
Basic sequencing skills (can tell you what happens next in a familiar storybook)
Draws a person with 3+ body parts

Receptive Language Milestones: how much your child is understanding of language:

Understands two-step directions (e.g. "get your shirt and put it in the hamper")
Understands contrasting concepts (e.g. big/small, hot/cold)
Recognized doorbell ringing or phone (demonstrated by pointing and showing excitement)
Understands simple "who," "where," and "what" questions
Can hear you and come when you call from another room (out of sight)
Can answer simple 'wh' questions about stories
Demonstrates understanding of the conversations going on at home, daycare, etc.

Expressive Language Milestones: length and complexity of language spoken
   General rule of thumb is a child's mean length of utterance (how much they say at a given time should equate with their age), for example, a 4-year-old will typically speak in 4 word utterances a majority of the time.

Complexity of a typical child's language from 3- to 4.5-year-olds

Language Complexity	Examples
1. Articles	1. A book, the book
2. Regular past tense (-ed endings on verbs)	2. She jumped, he laughed
3. Third person regular present tense	3. He swims, man brings

Social Communication Age Expectations (2–4-year-olds):

24–36 months

Engages in short dialogues
Verbally introduces and changes the topic
Expresses emotion
Begins to use language in an imaginative way
Relates own experiences
Begins to include descriptive details to enhance listeners understanding
Uses attention-getting words
Clarifies and asks for clarification
Uses politeness terms or markers
Begins to demonstrate adaptation of speech to different audience/listeners
Can deceive and detect deception
Understands that others may feel differently than themself
Follows rules
Shoes common but not daily schemes in play (e.g. doctor, shopping)
Uses embedded requests

3–4 years

Engages in longer dialogues
Anticipates next turn at talking
Terminates conversation; appropriately role-plays
Uses filers (e.g. "yeah" "okay") to acknowledge partners message
Begins code-switching and using simpler language when talking to very young
   children
Uses elliptical responses (e.g. "mommy went home, I didn't")
Requests permission
Begins using language for fantasies, jokes, and teasing
Makes conversational repairs when not understood and correct others
Infers information from a story and infers indirect meanings
Uses primitive narratives – events follow from central core
Uses inferences in stories

Point of Interest and Its Impact on Intervention

Piggybacking off the importance of knowing where a child is functioning is knowing "what makes a child tick." What I mean by that is what interests them, as an individual unlike anyone else. We acquire this knowledge from spending floor time with the child in a comfortable environment. The combination of knowing exactly where a child is in every aspect, developmentally, along with knowing their particular interests gives us an "in" and massive step ahead in attaining short- and long-term goals.

Therefore, while a first or even the first two to three sessions of therapy can seem like a 'wash' so to say, it can also be the most critical in therapy and intervention planning.

Now you may be thinking, just like I had when I started off years ago in the field, "Who has the time to check the milestones or make a note on small interests every child has, I only have 30 minutes with them from the time I walk in the door until the time I leave?" This is where the idea of The Protocol came to mind. I thought, wouldn't it be nice if I could literally check off the skills a child has, quickly, and have their current level of functioning highlighted to me alongside the area that is just in their area of intervention window? Understanding that certain skills can be gained in a session or two, we are talking about constantly moving the goalposts as a child progresses. Such a program would make every session easier along with the post-planning and writing a student's session notes. This also would help describe to parents the 'method behind the madness,' and why I am literally playing peek-a-boo and singing songs half of the session time.

From the problem came the eventual solution, The Protocol; no more wasted time scrolling through innumerable checklists and an easy calculable method to assist in daily treatment and progress monitoring.

The second part of the 'problem,' while attempting to set and make goals with children, is gaining their interest and intrigue in skilled therapy. This is where the second part of my point above comes in, figuring out what makes a child 'tick.' What are they specifically interested in that can really 'draw' them in and make them engaged in therapy.

This is where I inserted 'chicken scratch' onto my daily notes which read something like this 'plays with plastic bags,' 'likes to pop bubbles,' 'profound interest in animals,' and 'loves to lift the flap books.' To an untrained eye, this information on session notes may seem useless, however, I have found it to be profoundly useful during intervention with both children AND the adults that I have served over the years.

In summary, the merging of developmental milestones, the area of intervention, and the particular client interest has led to successful intervention. At the very least, I believe I have empowered my clients to feel good about themselves and make baby steps toward their goals. After all, we are not here to 'fix problems,' we work with living and breathing humans who each have their own interests and gifts to share with the world. We are here as a vehicle to help them reach their destinations.

I would like to expand upon this 'point of entry' further. What I am referring to when I speak about this is the ideas, stimuli, or interests that a client has. What makes them excited? What in their environment lights them up inside and brings a smile to their face? What do they like to explore or talk about?

You may be thinking, why does this matter when we are talking about setting goals and reaching those targets with our clients? The reason why this matters is, when you have a child (or adult) engaged in what you are presenting to them, they will be more willing and active participants in the actual learning of that new skill.

This is because, if we have motivation and engagement, results are easier to attain on both ends (therapist and client). Before anything else, a majority of our clients are aware that there is something 'not right' about their speech or language, it is a 'hard pill to swallow' that something is hard for you that may not be for others. In feeding off that innate *knowledge* that there is a deficit, we want our clients to feel empowered and good about themselves when they come to see us, or at least I do. Which is why most times during formal assessments I find myself apologizing for the length or the hardship of test completion and try to lighten the mood by asking my clients about themselves. If they cannot speak for themself, there is usually a family member or trusted confidant who can share little bits of information. This can yield, in my opinion, a successful therapist client interaction and relationship. I do find it to be a relationship, looking back on the now ten years of experience in the field there are times when I do think back on the clients and families I have served, wondering where they are, and how they are doing, like a long lost friend. I do know that, as long as I was able to make that connection which revolved around getting into their interests and world, I have succeeded, having completed my job as an 'Uber driver' to assist them in where they need to go for the next stage of their life.

To provide a personal example for this, I have never been good at math. In fact, I downright stunk in all math classes up to and including algebra. When math was mixed with letters I simply did NOT 'get it' whatsoever. I additionally was gifted with teachers who like to skip over steps and leave out practical applications of such concepts. I remember dreading math class so much that I would always seem to get sick before attending it from literally elementary school onwards. This was until I met a teacher who explained math in terms of application in my field. Of course, now we are talking about statistics and its analysis, but when I was able to see *visually* what this meant as far as where a child lands in relation to their peers, it clicked for me.

I can think of countless ways in which I use math to assist with practical applications (this obviously is impacted when I am in a restaurant and the tip calculation comes up or when I am calculating state taxes so I know how much I will have in the bank account at the end of the pay period). Needless to say, if I had a teacher who actually helped me connect the dots between my personal areas of interest and the mathematical concepts I needed to learn, perhaps I wouldn't have had such a hard time walking into those classes. Furthermore, I wouldn't still have this feeling of being "awful" at mathematical concepts.

The abovementioned 'point of interest' can carry over to various other applications with the clients we service. While 'vocabulary acquisition' seems so mundane and boring to most people, would it be boring if it is related to an area of personal interest? Let me recall a preschooler I had about six years ago in the field. I will call him Andre. Andre loved everything about animals. He would be found in the classroom with miniature zoo animals in his hands (often two at a time) which he loved to line up and carry with him everywhere. While Andre knew six or seven animals, he couldn't label many more. This is when I remembered a national geographic photo book I happened to have lying in my parents basement in a therapy pile. This book had everything, from sea lions to manta rays to sloths. Andre absolutely loved this book, and after two sessions he would "read" the book to me. I further was able to easily incorporate action questions to impart knowledge related to action words/verbs. Therapy sessions felt light, fun, and ease filled; Andre enjoyed coming and made great strides toward his long-term goals.

I would like to provide an example of utilization of this 'point of interest' as it pertains to some of the older students that I have served over the years. I used to work at a middle high school deep in Brooklyn, New York. This job took me one and a half hours to commute to and two subway train changes to get to, mind you. I had a student, we will call him Sebastian, who loved all things "trains." Sebastian had an obsession with Thomas the train, so much so that his Proloquo-to-go had an entire button with subsequent subcategories added to include the different characters. (Proloquo-to-go is an augmentative and alternative communication device, AAC). Sebastian's long-term goal was to utilize the device to formulate sentences, however, all that he wanted to do is to navigate to the page with Thomas the train and approximate the labels of the different characters. I found an opportunity to shape Sebastian's interest in Thomas the train, to subway trains and their consequent letters and colors, making his interests more functional. I pulled out a map of the New York City subway system and began listing the different lines with their subsequent colors and input them into his augmentative and alternative communication device (AAC). From that day forward, I was able to gain Sebastian's attention to ask and answer questions related to the subway lines throughout the city and its outer boroughs in the short sentence forms. We later shaped this interest to include certain food stores in the area that he would visit with his mother so he could identify the store and which line was closest to it. I had attained what we call personal 'buy in' to therapy. Sebastian loved to come to sessions and I even learned a thing or two about the local subway lines in the New York City area. Furthermore, we were able to make his device personally interesting to him and a means to 'talk about' areas that "lit him up inside."

Let me provide an example of the power of language as I pitched it to my older, middle school students in the Upper West Side of Manhattan. I cannot count the times that my 14-year-old group of 6th graders would saunter into the speech room stating they don't see the reason why they need to even write, let alone write an entire essay (to address written language deficits). There was seemingly no purpose for it in their minds. In the same five-minute interval, while they were settling into the speech room, they discussed their disagreement with the school uniform policy, and stated that the rules were pointless and they could still present themselves in a school-friendly way without ruining their personal style. Which, for those of you who have worked with middle schoolers know, their wardrobe mostly revolved around wearing hoodie sweatshirts. I stopped what I was doing and volunteered to work as a scribe for them, bulleting their seemingly 'valid' points and placing them on the classroom white board. Suddenly, everyone in the five-student group had a point to add. All along the way, I asked how I could write the sentence so it sounded like a lawyer who was representing them produced it. Kids were actively yelling out points, commenting and adding to their classmates; it was a fully engaged session. I stopped, and put a title to our work: Persuasive Essay: Students at MS 567 (made up for privacy sake) Pose an Amendment to School Uniforms. They were quiet for half a second and Shane retorted "we didn't write no essay," but I responded with, "You dictated an essay. How easy would it be to put all of this into something that resembled what your teacher is asking for?" "Pfft, we don't need more work, Miss L" stated another, to which I responded "Do you want Mr. V to listen to your uniform proposal?" To which there was a resounding 'yes' from the crowd with some slurs thrown in the mix. When they calmed down I said, "Well, writing is a form of expression. We seemed to write how we felt with desire for change easily here." After this session, I am happy to report that my 14-year-old group would run to me once a new essay was assigned in the classroom. I started every session off with a new "What do you want to say?" While these students are likely off to college or trade school at this point, I hope that they have found their voice through written language.

To provide yet another example, one of the speech-language pathologist assistants who was working under my supervision had a middle schooler who, quite literally, hated sessions with her. He would commence to threaten to call the state board to take away her license, to attend speech sessions with the hood up on his hoodie, and speak to her through the computer, even though they were in the same room as each other. When she came to be exasperated about how to possibly get through to this student, I asked a question that I often ask parents. "What is he interested in?" She paused and then commenced to explain how he loves politics and even debating political issues. "Interesting," I said. Then I asked about his goals and what he is able to do now. At this time, she stated that he was working on listening comprehension and written language (e.g. essay completion). She stated that he refused to listen to any books she presented to him and would not put a pen to paper. This is where I suggested we conduct our own research on local politics, both county and state. We were able to find associated and up-to-date articles, and we provided that as a baseline lesson plan to engage the student. While he was interested in spewing his opinions prior to the reading, turn taking was incorporated into the lesson and before we knew it, the student was stopping the speech-language pathologist assistant in the hall to tell her about up-to-date government events he had read on his own accord. When it came time to work on essay composition, we utilized the governor's model of writing (as a 'social story' or model of sorts) and 'ta-da,' the end result was a well thought out essay about an area of interest! Speech therapy superpower activated! For those of you who may not be aware of social stories, it is the utilization of a particular area of interest or superstar in which a child idolizes to provide appropriate social scripts or contexts of which the child needs to model to interact with others in a socially acceptable way. I will place a resource at the end of this portion for your review and further inquiry.

Now some of you may be thinking that it's easy working with elementary children, they love to play games and talk about Star Wars characters, how do I interest a 14-year-old? To which again, I go back to observing and asking about what they do in their spare time. Let me provide an example here. I had a student, Bobby, let's call him, while I was working in the New York City public schools. Bobby presented as a hyperactive 13-year-old, tall and wiry, with so much energy that he would often be found fumbling to keep his pants up on his thin frame. He spoke "a mile a minute" and would constantly be mentioning his love of Fortnight. For those of you who are not familiar with Fortnight, it is a video game in which you can compete and play with others internationally. I later came to know that Bobby was a well-established Fortnight player online and had won some smaller 'tournaments.' Now, I was in my mid-thirties at the time, far from a 'hip teen.' However, I knew that there was something 'there' with Bobby's specific interest. To which I signed onto the favored Newsela and found a leveled reader related to gaming. (Newsela is an online platform available in the United States which provides 'leveled readers' which are based on a certain child's reading ability). This article may have been the entryway to engage Bobby in our speech sessions. Of course, like other middle schoolers, his goals were related to written language and reading comprehension, however, he met these goals easily with a stimulus that was of paramount interest to him. Suddenly he went from a student who couldn't put two words together on a paper to dictating a full essay (with assistance) about the infamous Fortnight star at the time, Bugha?

In this circumstance, I figured out where Bobby was currently functioning, putting three to four words together on a sheet of paper and barely able to attend to an age-leveled reader; and advanced him to writing paragraphs and an eventual essay on an area of interest. Therefore, the merging of current functioning level, intervention level, and personal interests came together to yield a personal speech success story.

To this day I think about Bobby, who is now probably about to graduate high school. I hope that he continues to share his enthusiasm for the gaming world, and he will think about the fun times we had during our speech sessions sharing and 'writing' about areas of interest. I hope I was able to help him find his "written voice."

Now, I will pay devil's advocate here for a second. I have and still work with adults on an on-call capacity in the subacute and assisted living facilities, and, as you might imagine, I have come across a multitude of 'push back' from clients on therapy or even accepting my entry into their rooms to glean insight into their case. However, it has almost always served me to just "check in" and have a conversation with a client upon their first arrival asking them to speak about themselves and further following up with active listening questions to establish a healthy rapport. Let's face it, who doesn't like to be asked about themselves? This is often an immediate buy-in to therapy with the older ages as they feel heard, and they have a connection to the facility they are residing in temporarily. The second part of this is it requires their active consent and buy-in from the get-go which makes them feel in control when their health, and likely, other areas of their lives do not feel as such.

I want you to think back to the clients in which you have built the strongest bonds with over the years. What have you done differently to set up those working relationships? I could beg to guess that they are based on the connection and engagement with another's interests which can serve as an invaluable facet to successful therapy.

In summary, identification of a client's interests serves us astronomically well in providing therapy which is uplifting and exciting for both our clients and ourselves. After all, I have always found it so interesting to learn about new topics that could seem mundane but are not to someone else. This is where perspective taking and intuition come in handy as a clinician.

It also never ceases to amaze me just how creative I can get while lesson planning a session with a child whose interests vary vastly from my own.

Behavior and Development

We have all experienced this, a young child whose only interest is in dumping toys out of bins or pushing food off the table. To an onlooker, the child is 'causing a ruckus' or maybe even difficult. This is where the awareness of typical development can glean insights into a child's behavior. I have found this particularly helpful when treating a child whose area of development is in the more primary stages as mentioned in the above examples. What I am proposing is that with the particular milestones (e.g. "peek-a-boo" or "cause effect" interest), we are provided with a jumping off point to begin intervention that actively engages a child right away.

I had mentioned before that my interest in psychology mainly stemmed from the question of 'why' behind human behavior. I would like to propose melding this with speech-language pathology and the potential of assigning some meaning behind the 'why' in children's behavior, suggesting that most behavior can have communicative intent if the basic cognitive functioning is there. What if behavior was communication? Behavior as a means to communicate for those who have no other way to get their point across?

After working with preschool District 75 students (students who are in the special needs preschool) you almost expect a tantrum at the beginning or end of a speech session. When I started to reflect back from the antecedent and behavior (what happened that preceded the behavior), I drew a parallel quickly. Times of transition are particularly hard for our children, in general. Imagine this, you are having a lovely time hanging out with friends when suddenly someone turns off the show you are both watching, or you are in the middle of singing a great jam when the radio tunes out. What is the innate feeling you have? Is it frustration, anger perhaps, sadness? All of these feelings would be completely justified for us to feel; therefore, why are we surprised when our children experience them as well? Perhaps it is because a vast majority of them do not yet have the words to express how they are feeling. Angry? Throw the book. Sad? Drop to the floor. Unable to express those feelings? Scream and cry. This is where functional communication comes in as arguably our greatest superpower.

I can refer back to my work as a personal aide in a special needs preschool in North Jersey, the beginning of the summer marked the first time these preschoolers were in a school setting. Naturally, there were tantrums, a ton of toys being strewn across the room, food pushed onto the floor – the whole gambit of behaviors. However, as I noticed that with collaboration between the speech-language pathologist, the head teacher, and the aides, the behaviors decreased as the students' functional communication increased. There is a strong correlation between behavior and communication.

From a pre-speech standpoint, I had noticed this prior to my return to academics for my masters when I took a job at a well-known daycare center. For privacy purposes, we will call it Rivland Academy. I was hired as a class teacher to help with the T-2 classroom (toddler), who was having a "biting issue." Being always up for a challenge, I gladly accepted the position and was pointed in the direction of the core perpetrator (who had 'started it all'). It only took me about 30–60 minutes to figure out the 'biting problem.' There was no facilitator to assist with concepts such as sharing and turn taking and thus came out the "choppers." I also noted that the 'key perpetrator' was rather slow in her move to bite others, meaning, easily caught if under a more watchful eye. I also observed that the 'key perpetrator' was slow in her attempts to bite others, making it easy to intervene if closely monitored. This further highlighted the connection between behavior and communication, even in a setting where the children were, for all intents and purposes, typically developing. After guided intervention (namely utilization of functional baby sign and replacement of behavior with modeling), I advanced to other classrooms in Rivland Academy for my 'skills.' I put the skills in parenthesis here, as I was just correlating behavior with communicative intent. Needless to say, it was my first pre-speech experience with the correlation between such principles. Since, it has served me, to this day, when a child has a behavioral outburst in the universal preschool classrooms that I serve, I have been able to acknowledge and correlate it with a communicative intent.

Of course, we know that just sharing that we are upset will likely not change the outcome – cue, cleaning up the toys, and walking back to the classroom – however, we are able to express our thoughts and feelings which can sometimes help to dispel them. Suddenly, words and expressing ourselves have more purpose than simply stating requests – but on commenting or even displaying refusal/rebuttal. As you will see in the subsequent speech and language milestones, there is a part of development when it is expected for children to refuse and question directives given to them by authority.

Overview of Language Scaffolding and Modeling Procedures

I would be remiss if I introduced the concept of The Protocol and did cover intervention methods that I use day in and out so much so that it became hard to label them at times! I think the first time in years that I labeled intervention procedures was when I was observing a personal favorite speech-language pathologist assistant (SLPA) who I have. For those of you that are on the east coast of the United States and may not be aware of this profession, it is known as speech-language pathologist assistant. They have an undergraduate in communication sciences and disorders and conduct treatment under the purview of a licensed speech-language pathologist. I digress; I noticed that during my observation sessions I was literally writing all of the treatment-based methods she was using. My document sounded something like this: "Fill-in-blank, MC (multiple choice), and binary choice offered to improve word finding/vocabulary acquisition as mod (moderate) VV (verbal visual) cues." I was so used to writing session notes related to the amount of cueing (e.g. mod VVT cues – moderate verbal, visual, tactile) that I seemed to be on autopilot with the rest of the methods that we employ daily as speech interventionists. However, it was a breath of fresh air to visually and physically note these interventions utilized during skilled sessions.

Therefore, this chapter may be an accolade to one of my top speech-language pathologist assistants who I supervise! I will not name names, but know that I have your model in the back of my mind while I share the treatment and intervention methods that you have utilized in every single session I have observed you.

This is a time where a speech-pathologist provides an overview of the research-backed methods which are generally based on learning theories which are tried and true. Such methods as recasting, scaffolding, and modeling are employed and utilized in almost every session we provide to our clients (of all ages). Without diving into a clinical methods class, I will affirm that having personally researched additional methods behind some of the psychology masterminds (e.g. Vygotsky) certain methodologies were discussed (namely scaffolding).

You may be thinking to yourself, why is she reviewing such methods in this protocol? There is a method behind this 'madness' namely because these methods act as facilitators to take our children from where they are currently to where they are going. In graduate school, I recall an entire course on this, namely clinical methods and procedures. The amazing part of this is that after years in the field we use the abovementioned methods without even thinking about them. However, when they are utilized appropriately, they are paramount in assisting a child in skills acquisition and mastery.

I will attach a 'language scaffolding and modeling checklist' to the back of this chapter for quick reference. I had actually produced this for a parent workshop I hosted in the middle of the COVID-19 lockdown in 2020, with layman's terms in mind (to assist in description for our non-speechie counterparts). While I included these in a parent training course, I myself found it helpful to review all the methods that are utilized throughout the course of a session. If not for my own knowledge, however, these methods can arguably be described as a 'skilled' service, as speech-pathologists (and some special education teachers) are trained in the belowmentioned methods.

First of all, I would like to review the language modeling procedures in brief. These are described as recurring pictures or examples of a target. They are especially beneficial as the noted 'reoccurring' or repetition which is embedded in the method, as we learn through targeted repetition of interventions. When we speak about a prompt or cue it's the minimal amount of support, or clues needed to evoke the correct response. This could look like minimal verbal cues (e.g. repetition × 1 of the direction), or minimal verbal/visual cues (e.g. one verbal direction with gesture).

The second language modeling strategy that we utilize almost on auto-pilot, is recasting. This is when you take what a child says, but repeat it with accuracy. This can work for articulation errors (e.g. child – "big wabbit!"; therapist – yes, that's a big white rabbit); grammatical errors (e.g. child – "two mouses!"; therapist – "I see two brown MICE!"

The final language modeling technique I want to discuss is called successive approximation. In this approach, the clinician helps the child develop more complex responses by building on simpler ones the child already knows. For example, if you ask a child to wash their hands, and they walk to the sink and stand by it, you reinforce that action. Then, as you guide them through turning on the water, and they reach for the soap, you acknowledge that they are gradually mastering the complete hand-washing routine through these successive steps.

The easiest way to describe some of these language scaffolding methods is in the context of an early intervention speech session, where we are stimulating and further expanding upon language. I will place 'fill in the blanks' along with expectant pause, as I feel they go 'hand in hand' so to say. Fill in the blanks are when you model part of the utterance and pause (expectant pause) for the child to complete the rest of it. Typically this is our model of the first part of the utterance (e.g. 'row, row, row, your ...) waiting for the child to verbally approximate 'boat.' This strategy is best utilized with rote or routine tasks/activities that you know the child knows like the back of their hand. An example is a familiar song that Mommy sings with their child or a familiar book (e.g. 'I love my white shoes. I love my white ...-shoes). What makes fill-in-the-blanks along with expectant pause so effective? Number one, our children KNOW the answer, and it further gives them confidence to fill in that blank, plus they have this burning need to complete the sequence. It builds on confidence and sets them up for success.

The second teaching method which comes most inherently to a lot of the speech-language pathologists I have worked with are gestures and facial expressions. Think about it this way, when you walk into a room and see a friend, how do you inherently act? Do you smile and wave? We often utilize these 'non-verbal' communication methods to demonstrate our feelings and excitement toward a person and/or event. This is where direct modeling of these gestures and expressions, with over accentuation, is particularly helpful when our child is learning language. Going on a walk with a child, point and provide exclamations (Whoa!! Look! I see ... dog). To provide another example, when I started providing early intervention in the homes in the Flatiron district of Manhattan I would walk around with a large Hulken bag. My children knew that was the location of all the 'goodies' so to say. And I would take it off my back, making an exaggerated exclamation "woof!, boom" as I put it on the ground in front of them. I would often shake it and shrug my shoulders while asking, 'what should I do?' This is where I was able to scaffold a functional 'open' sign and eventual functional verbal request "open bag please!" to incite functional communication and requests.

The next area of language scaffolding is preparatory sets. I think these are most relevant when I have worked with children in the academic sector, while I am preparing them for higher-level concepts they will be taught in class. Having worked in a middle school in the upper west side, my motto quickly became 'help them in their academics' do not add to their current workload. Mostly this came from the sixth graders telling me "Ohh man, don't you give us more work, Miss LoPresti!" At this moment I set out to really 'kill it' at collaboration and ask the teachers for sneak peeks of upcoming projects and lessons. I still remember being given this social studies lesson to prep my eighth graders for, I was able to find the associated NewsELA article (for those of you who are not familiar with this, it is a program which modifies readers based on a child's ability, and it basically scaffolds them based on word count, complexity, etc.). The group and I reviewed the articles fully, for over 2 weeks – brainstorming arguments, making our own personal notes, etc. Finally, the day came where the lesson was taught and my students had the floor to share or comment. I made sure to be standing outside the room quietly so I could see if they were able to 'share their thoughts and analysis'; Benji, one of my students raised his hand emphatically and shared the meaning of a vocabulary word in the reader and HIS thoughts on the article. Everyone in the class was quiet, the teacher beamed and acknowledged him, and his peers sat there collaborating with him. I think this taught me the value of an appropriate 'prep-set,' and how it can really assist in adding value while setting our children up for success.

Let's talk about phonemic cues. This is when a therapist provides the first sound/sound cluster to assist with a child's retrieval of the correct response. This can also assist with adults who have anomia (word-finding deficits). An example would be when asking a child what city we are in, after a pause saying "New ... Y" providing them the phonemic cue for them to start the word correctly. I like to think that this method can assist with 'tip of the tongue' syndrome, when you just KNOW the word you are looking for but you can't seem to retrieve it, it's an added 'cue' to assist with finding that word in your mental catalog.

Binary choice is a method I have utilized for both children and adults as their statistical chances of getting the right answer are infinitely higher. This also can assist when a client knows the answer but they cannot retrieve it or the options need to be super simplified. Binary, meaning two, so it is simply providing a choice of two. I have utilized this countless times when providing an option for snacks, when working on feeding goals, e.g., do you want the goldfish or pretzels? Oftentimes I utilize either a visual (picture) of the items, or the actual items themselves. I will accept a simple gesture (point), sign (e.g. give me), or verbal request/label (e.g. goldfish). Again, a method to set our clients up for communicative success.

I like to utilize the next scaffolding method after I have completed a task with a child in their home to 'describe' to their parent or nanny 'how' we did such a task. An example would be making soap snow. What is this, you may ask? Well, it is basically a hair conditioner with baking soda which yields a cold substance that is much like snow. Of course, when I have made such a 'craft' with my early intervention babies before, there has been a visual recipe card accompanying the directions simplified, so we can 'follow directions' and the child can help ME complete the task with the result of home snow. The summarization prompt is used when I ask the child to "tell mommy HOW we made snow!" I will often show them the picture recipe card so they can successfully retell the steps needed to complete the activity we have completed together. This way they can 'tell mommy' how to make snow at home themselves.

The last language scaffolding method I want to review here is perhaps most apparent to my speechies who are working on listening comprehension and pre-literacy skills. The good ole 'comprehension questions' of which we utilize every time we are reading a story using the dialogic method. Reading /Pete the cat/? Who is in this story? What is he wearing? What happened? All questions, with associated visual cues set our children up for success, when asking further inquiry questions about a story. This method is utilized during play in a preschool classroom, who are we playing with? While pointing to a classmate. What are we making? While gesturing toward the pretend spaghetti. You get the point here! This does eventually build on itself so that when we ask our children 'what happened on the playground' they can utilize recall and their vocabulary to share an event that happened in the past (cue, higher-level language concepts here).

Language Scaffolding and Modeling Checklist

Language Scaffolding: *Techniques used to facilitate language and thought!*

Strategy	Definition
Fill-in-the-blanks	Model part of utterance and pause for the child to complete the sentence
Gestures/facial expressions	Use of natural gestures (point, shrug) and facial expressions (smile, surprise) to demonstrate meaning behind words
Prep sets	Showing your child HOW to express an idea
Expectant pause	Asks a question and then waits/pauses while looking to your child to respond (verbal turn-taking)
Phonemic cues	Adult gives first sound/sound cluster to give child clues to the correct response
Binary choices	Two options for child to choose between (giving child options)
Summarization prompt	Adult re-creates steps in an activity they did together
Comprehension questions	Asking more information than your child is giving ("wh" questions)

Language Modeling: *Reoccurring pictures or examples of the target!*

Strategy	Definition
Recasting	Taking what your child said and changing it slightly to make it more correct
Prompt or Cue	Providing the minimal clue sufficient to evoke the correct response
Successive approximation	Shaping new, more complex responses from simpler responses already in your child's repertoire (e.g. asking what color of an item labeled, or how many ...)

Non-English Speaker Considerations

I would be remiss if I did not review the importance of assessment and further intervention being conducted in a child's first spoken language. A child's first language is that language which is spoken and modeled to them in the home. While a lot of schools in the United States are primarily English speaking, the children that I have been referred to over the years are already receiving primary English instruction. This comes from the age-old "issue" when administration refers a child whose native language is not English for an evaluation by a monolingual speech-pathologist. The monolingual speech-pathologist that I am referring to is myself! Mono means only fluent in one language.

I cannot count the amount of lengthy discussions we received in graduate school regarding assessments needing to be in a child's first native language. For this reason, I always inquire about background history and ask about what language a child is spoken to in the home before accepting an evaluation. Nevertheless, there is almost always push-back; stating a therapist is not available who speaks the native language or that they can have a translator for the assessment. In these cases, I will often quote ethical and best practice concerns and considerations and require they attempt to locate an appropriate provider.

However, there have been spare cases in which I have had to complete an initial assessment on a child whose language is not English speaking. You may be asking, how in the world can you do such a thing? Well, to start off, my report is riddled with statements up to and including the fact that the child's native language is (insert language), and therefore English assessments cannot be utilized to determine disorder – only difference, which is expected for an English language learner. The second portion I do want to note, there are many facets about language that are universal. For example, a child is in the room and mom asks them to sit in a chair and look at the screen; this direction can be given in any language, however, if a child is able to follow the directive IN their native language, this is telling.

Another area that I look at is the mean length of utterance – listening to the interactions between parent and child and asking the parent what was said can glean the length and even complexity of language utilized. While I would like to say that such informal assessments can only be utilized as a mere screener, a general gist of a child's current speech and language abilities can be ascertained. This is where the most important questions are asked in which I can glean how far off a child is from where they should be developmentally speaking. Questions such as, does she follow simple 2 step directions, how rich is her vocabulary, can they answer 'wh' questions, can you understand what they are saying?

I had a recent referral for a 5-year-old, Cantonese speaking little girl. The SST team (student support team) had provided me with an initial 'formal' evaluation by a local hospital. The concerns were "understanding of directions and language learning." I had come to realize that the PLS (Preschool Language Scale) was administered in English, her non-native language and the standard scores were provided. If I were sharing this story with some of my clinical fellows I would ask them to point out the two errors they noticed immediately. Which would be utilization of standardized scores on a test normed on English speakers and a further formal assessment administered in a second language. I digress. After I requested a Cantonese speaking provider and the district was unable to locate one I agreed to provide a screen within reason. Emily was an energetic little girl, who had "boundless" energy. I was able to gain an informal functional language sample through assistance of her mother, who spoke to Emily in Cantonese. I told her mother that while I would be speaking to her in English, I asked her to translate to her daughter in her native language. Over the course of the hour-long session, Emily was able to follow multi-step directions, engage in a five to six word length of utterance with her mother, and further label items in a picture book in either English or Cantonese (if she couldn't find the English word for it). While my observations could not prove a language ability in the child's first language of Cantonese, it did provide valuable insight to bring to the student support team. The insight was Emily is an English language learner, she is seemingly proficient in her first language of Cantonese but is still learning English skills. This may appear to a monolingual teacher as a child who has receptive and potential expressive language deficits, however, children who are learning two languages at once (bilinguals) do experience lags in one language over the other. Furthermore, the mother and I developed a nice relationship during the observation and informal evaluation as I was able to share what I look out for in my English language speakers and check if Emily had these skills in Cantonese.

Let me provide another case study to demonstrate the intricacies of children who speak English as their second language (or ESL). I was referred to consult a child, let's call him Adan, whose native language was not English. The child was Gujarati speaking, both parents were fluent in the home and the child was instructed in English in the school. The consult came from a guidance counselor asking about typical articulation development and how to tackle the child's articulation errors if English is their second language. I asked the guidance counselor to let me know the sounds that were in error so I can glean some insight behind the complexity of the sound production and compare that to the child's age. The child's errors were in the /d/ and /g/ sounds. Off the bat I thought, these sounds are earlier acquisitioning, Adan should definitely have these, but in order to follow due diligence I sent a quick note to a graduate school professor who speaks the language. He referred me to the East Asian ASHA interest group, however when I did not receive a response I asked him, does Gujarati have the /d/ and /g/ sounds in the language? He responded with a resounding yes and followed this up by stating that they are (like their English counterpart) simpler sounds to produce, from a co-articulation standpoint. This is when I responded to the guidance counselor that an evaluation referral for such speech sound errors, although in a child's second language, would be beneficial.

All this to say, when there are instances where a child is not able to be assessed in their native language, there are ethical and culturally sound methods to utilize while attempting to provide best care and services. This is where a general knowledge of norms in not only English but other languages would prove beneficial in our field. With that being said, I would personally and professionally welcome evidence and collaboration across languages to further expand our knowledge across languages.

Literacy across Ages

After re-reading my personal journey as a speech-language pathologist I noted a particular pattern in my interventions which I feel is important to note in this text. This is the embedding of literacy in therapy sessions, across ages. I particularly enjoy the utilization of literacy in sessions as it serves as a 'visual language' of sorts to our clients. Besides the actual words on the page, the pictures in associated books, and/or newspapers can additionally serve as a point of reference between our clients and ourselves (as speech-language pathologists).

Whether it be during a preschool speech session, early intervention, school age or even adult and geriatric; I utilize text as a means to connect and provide a 'point of reference' for the intervention. While my babies enjoy looking at simple books with photographs, my teenagers and adults enjoy looking at the newspaper or other print to remain 'up to date' on the happenings.

To expand beyond the importance of utilizing an all-encompassing therapy tool during intervention; a newspaper can be utilized to assist with executive functioning skills with children who are of middle school age through adulthood. To list just a few of the executive functioning skills: orientation to time and date as well as location (which is provided at the top of the newspaper), planning (when referencing the 'television guide' or activities in the local newspaper), and working and short-term memory (with a visual to aide in retention and recall of questions associated with recent events).

I will touch on the concept of Dialogic Reading in the chapter that covers 'Brown's Morphological and Syntactic Development,' as this method of 'reading' with my clients, across ages; has assisted greatly in developing daily therapy materials that are relevant and targeting the skills which are listed in The Protocol. While I do not explicitly mention utilization of pre-literacy or literacy-based materials for interventions in every consequential chapter, it is a valid resource for not only assisting in language acquisition and reacquisition, but also as a means to 'connect' more deeply with my clients while establishing and grow rapport.

A Note on Executive Functioning

In the upcoming chapters, I will mention executive functioning well over a dozen times, which has led me to add some context here, as a teaser of sorts. In thinking back on my original draft of The Protocol, I actually had an 'executive functioning' chapter that I wanted to include but did not have the time nor bandwidth to include it in my original submission. Therefore, you will attain my 'take' on our role, as speech-language pathologists and interventions as they relate to our scope and practice with clients of ALL ages.

As defined, executive functioning skills are noted to be "higher-level cognitive skills" entail the following areas of cognitive processing and functioning: "working memory, inhibitory control, cognitive flexibility, metacognition, fluid/abstract reasoning skills, complex problem solving, as well as advanced Theory of Mind skills." It is understood that a person's executive functioning is dependent on core cognitive functions working together such as attention, processing speed, and memory (ASHA, 2024). As you will note in upcoming chapters, many of these abovementioned 'skills' are listed in the developmental norm chapters.

Examples of executive functioning deficits in the children and adults we service can include difficulty with organization of their binder or locker for school, inability to complete assignments on time, difficulty navigating social situations as well as managing their own medication administration (this is particularly a huge one for the adult population).

From a core and foundational language learning perspective, attention and lack thereof can greatly impact the results we attain in a given session with children who exhibit fleeting attention. It is hard to learn a new skill if anything you are interacting with is momentary at best. This is where purposeful intervention ON gaining and increasing a child's attention is imperative. Devices such as 'light up wands' or 'jigglers' have been utilized in the past to assist in gaining and sustaining children's attention.

After a child (or adult rather) has attention then you can address 'working memory' and further 'short-term memory' deficits. I cannot count the amount of times I have been in attendance to an Individualized Education Plan, and the psychologist has identified executive functioning deficits in the area of memory and shifts the intervention onto the speech-pathologists domain. This is where we utilize our compensatory strategy methods to assist in teaching children ways to retrieve and recall information provided to them (e.g. write it down, chunking, pneumonic devices, etc.). The same strategies which I list here are appropriate across ages.

I hope to input this subheading into the introduction test to place "in the back of your mind" when you are planning a course of intervention with any client (from babyhood through adulthood). The abovementioned skills are foundational to the skills we teach in the following subsets of our field.

References

Center on the Developing Child at Harvard University. (2020, March 24). *Executive Function & Self-regulation.* https://developingchild.harvard.edu/science/key-concepts/executive-function/

Mcleod, S. (2024, February 1). Albert Bandura's social learning theory in psychology. *Simply Psychology.* https://www.simplypsychology.org/bandura.html

3 Piaget's Stages

To provide background on Piaget's Stages, Jean Piaget was famous for his "theories which were related to changes in cognitive development that spans from infancy through adulthood. Piaget believed that cognitive development occurred at the intersection of nature (innate capabilities) and nurture (the child's environment)" (McLeod, 2018). Piaget's theories are broken down into four stages which represent cognitive abilities and comprehension of the world. Beyond his theories, Piaget suggested that active exploration and interaction with one's environment assist in shaping an individual's cognitive development. With each stage, a child develops and constructs a "mental model of the world, or schema" (McLeod, 2018).

Since this portion of The Protocol only includes four stages, it is crucial to dive into each stage in more detail to assist in developing appropriate interventions based on the stage in which your child is performing. What I appreciate about Piaget's stages is that, while there are 'typical ages' of acquisition, these are flexible and are all determined on the cross between nature and nurture based on each child as an individual. Therefore, bear with me as I describe each stage in more detail before providing the checklist for this intervention area. Piaget proposed that intelligence develops through a series of stages, all fueled by a child's internal world.

The *sensorimotor stage* is the first cognitive developmental stage, as described by Piaget. The sensorimotor stage is when we see children banging and shaking toys and putting them in their mouths. Sensorimotor is the stage where children learn about their environment through their senses and hands-on exploration. What it looks like is a child who is 'mouthing everything' in their environment. While it is typical for a 3- to 6-month-old child to mouth everything, I have also seen children close to age 5 exploring their environment in the same way. Sensorimotor is the age where children develop object permanence – the knowledge that just because something is out of sight does not mean it has disappeared completely. Object permanence is essential and can speak to separation anxiety for a child from

DOI: 10.4324/9781003491842-3

a parent, if this is not developed. Self-recognition is also developed at this stage, which is the understanding of themselves as a different entity from their parent, peer, etc. At this stage, children realize that their actions can cause reactions from the world around them (e.g. if I jump up onto the table, mommy will run after me). Representational play develops later in this stage; an example would be a child taking a toy car and driving it on the ground or making noises associated with a vehicle. How is this a significant building block to assist in developing other areas of speech and language development? To advance a child to a more cognitively and linguistically advanced stage, a clinician must meet the child where they are currently developing. For a child exploring through mouthing and banging, the best way is to introduce these simple concepts through play at this age. An example of intervention would be pounding a ball, rolling balls between each other, banging spoons on the table next to the baby, and imitating vocal play.

The second Piagetian stage of development is known as the *preoperational stage*. The primary characteristic of this stage is that a child will begin to acquire the ability to represent the world internally through language and mental images. They start to think about things symbolically, which perfectly lends itself to language acquisition, as this speaks to making one thing (e.g. the word 'cookie') stand for something other than itself (e.g. an actual cookie). This is the stage where our children expand on their expressive language skills. They realize a word has an actual meaning for an object or concept. Children are egocentric at this age, meaning they do not yet have a theory of mind and assume that everyone else sees the world as they do. Children in this stage of development also demonstrate what is known as animism, which is the tendency for a child to think that non-living objects have feelings (e.g. thinking their dolls live their own lives when they leave the room). Toward the end of the preoperational stage, a child will begin to enjoy imaginative play. At the end of the preoperational stage, interventions can include collaborative talk-alouds during pretend play in the kitchen or with their dolls. As a refresher, 'talk alouds' are also known as narration of actions or events we are doing AS we are doing them. An example of a 'talk aloud' would be "Dolly is tired, she's yawning, she's going to get ready for bed. What should she do first?"

Piaget's third stage is known as the *concrete operational stage*. Children in this stage of development are still literal and concrete in their way of thinking; however, they can develop a sense of logic. At this stage, children struggle with abstract or hypothetical concepts. Many of our children who are on the autism spectrum have a hard time figuring out the what-ifs outside of the prescribed events of any given day on the way to school. Children at this stage begin to understand the concept of conservation (e.g. the amount of water can be the same despite the size of the cup it is in). At this stage, children develop a theory of mind and begin to understand that their thoughts are unique. An example of a child who may have difficulty at this stage of development would not know when they said something seemingly hurtful to a friend when they thought they were giving facts. An area of growth for this stage would include pragmatic interventions (social skills training) to develop this area further.

Piaget's fourth and final stage is known as *formal operational*. Typically, this stage begins when a child is around 11. Formal operational is when children acquire the ability to think abstractly, combine and classify items sophisticatedly, and have the capacity for higher-order reasoning. In layperson's terms, this allows children to understand politics and science fiction and engage in scientific reasoning. Abstract ideas can include mathematical division and fractions. These are higher-level language functions, including following an argument without considering examples and dealing with hypothetical problems and solutions (e.g. 'What if our car broke down?'). Hypothetical problems and situations correlate directly to problem-solving and other executive functioning skills that are quite obviously more advanced life skills where our children can benefit from explicit training. For a specific example which is arguably academic based, these are the students who we are assisting with essay and written language composition. In the formal operational stage, we are drawing on logical conclusions and collecting data to support our assumptions.

As you can see, where a child falls in their development related to Piaget's stages can vastly influence the appropriate intervention in speech and the formal classroom. Piaget's stages can also assist with functional goal development, ensuring that even the long-term goals are within the child's current stage (if they are in the sensorimotor stage) or one stage above (if they are performing at the end of the sensorimotor stage and are interested in pretend play). Regarding speech and language intervention, Piaget's stages can embody the concept of "meet a child WHERE they are currently functioning." With The Protocol, you can utilize their current stage to bridge them to subsequently more challenging stages to approximate age-appropriate levels more closely.

Causes of Deficiencies

As you have noticed, there is a very clear distinction between advancing stages of Piaget. This can result in some of our clients not ever reaching the higher-level cognitive functioning skills (e.g. formal operational and abstract thinking). Such a reason for a child with deficiencies in such areas can range from intellectual disabilities, to ASD's (autism spectrum disorders), to other syndromes that impact a child's concept of the world as they grow.

Sample Milestone Score with Interventions

Anna was a 6-month-old who could be found in her high chair banging items on the top of the high chair. She exhibited typical sensorimotor stage behavior, and she banged her rattle and utensils on the high chair, brought everything to her mouth, and liked peek-a-boo. Apart from the 'peek-a-boo' games, she did not exhibit joint attention (or engagement with caregivers' eyes).

Zone of Development: Transitioning from higher-level sensorimotor to preoperational stage

Intervention: Encourage direct imitation through banging and shaking a rattle, emphasizing exaggerated noises and actions like "tap tap tap" and expressing surprise with "uh-oh!" As the rattle drops, use pointing and gestural cues to help the child track its location, even when it's not in direct view.

With the utilization of meeting Anna at her current stage and interest and expanding on it through knowledge of core concepts to be mastered where she is, it is easier to bridge the gap between where Anna is and the next area of targeted intervention.

Important Collaborative Considerations

Collaboration with special educators and instructional interventionists is vital to assisting a child progress toward the more advanced stages of Piaget. Discrete trials and training in certain skills (e.g. object permanence) with assistance of another professional (e.g. an applied behavioral analyst therapist) can greatly assist in compliance toward learning new skills that could prove difficult to some children. I have observed early intervention ABA therapy sessions where repetition, distinct trials, and cause-and-effect are explicitly taught. While it has been suggested that such training is 'rigid' in nature, I have seen firsthand how it has greatly assisted my children who are more insular in attaining advanced skills. If we learn skills through 'doing' an actual action, then repetition of such action can glean results.

Preferred Methods and Procedures

When we are talking about important skills for a child to acquire, a combination of both naturalistic play and interaction AND distinct training can assist in bridging the gap between deficit and more typical functioning.

Piaget's 4 stages of Cognitive Development

Stage	Description	Goal of Stage	Age	Acquired? If So Which Portion (All, Some)
Sensorimotor stage	Learns through moving and exploring environment (object permanence, self-recognition, deferred imitation, and representational play) Emergence of symbolic function	Object permanence (requires ability to form mental representation – schema of object) toward end of stage use one object to stand for another Language begins b/c its used to represent objects and feelings	Birth – 18/24 months	
Preoperational stage	Internally represent world through language/mental imagery; demonstration of animism	Symbolic thought	2–7 years	
Concrete operational stage	Logical thinking about concrete events; understand concept of conservation (certain properties remain the same); think more about how others think and feel	Logical thought	7–11 years	
Formal operational stage	Can deal with abstract ideas (e.g. fractions); follow an argument without specific examples; deal with hypothetical problems	Scientific reasoning	Adolescence to adults	

Naturalistic play in this context: I am referring to following a child's lead to see what interests them naturally. Distinct training in this context: it is necessary to provide hand–over-hand instruction, or maximal verbal/visual and tactile cues to demonstrate a certain skill. An example would be demonstration of object permanence by assisting the baby to move the tissue paper off the dolly through hand-over-hand interaction; you are demonstrating an object is still in existence even though it is out of sight.

Therefore, I have utilized a combination approach to assist children in advancing toward Piaget's later acquired stages, melding a naturalistic approach with explicit skills training to glean results.

As far as important interventions to consider regarding Piaget's later stages, such as the concrete and formal operational, the stimuli should be age and cognition appropriate. For example, I had a number of children in my specialized music school who performed unmeasurably "off the charts" related to their cognitive abilities as measured in psychological tests, however, they could not figure out how to appropriately start or end a conversation with a peer. This particular population would be completely offended if I presented them with examples that included a more 'juvenile' social story (such as Paw Patrol pups), however, if I shared a story about, let's say Mozart, interest would be piqued. As you may notice, age or rather maturity level has a great impact on the treatment stimuli and interventions that are utilized.

Formal operational skills are arguably easily applicable in both the academic sector and personal or home-areas. An example of the formal operational intervention could be as simple as programming a child's augmentative alternative device (AAC) with the exact address of their parent's home and their school name which can be utilized in a case of emergency or they are separated from caregivers. Another example of intervention in Piaget's formal operational stage would be the collaboration during a science lab or experiment, in which students have to complete questions as they relate to scientific reasoning (such as testing a hypothesis).

Reference

McLeod, S.A. (2018, June 6). Jean Piaget's theory of cognitive development. *Simply Psychology*. www.simplypsychology.org/piaget.html

4 Parten's Social Stages of Play

Anyone who is of the same generation as I am could recall the familiar jingle (in the United States) – "I don't wanna grow up, I'm a toy's r' us kid." Of course, it was one of the major toy stores in the United States in the 80's who literally pitched 'toys' as a method to staying young and playing all day. I used to personally love that jingle, and that store. Even now, I do have many days where I feel "I played today." For those of us who have been in the field, and studied child development and their interaction in the environment, it is understandable that play is a 'serious' business of learning for our children. This is the way in which our children explore the world around them and provide 'mental schemas' as the great psychologists would say. While we do play with children, our methods are forever based on expanding their play skills and abilities. This is where guided knowledge and further intervention can assist in pinpointing the gap between where a child is functioning and where they should be based on age-appropriate peers.

After working in this field for a while, I get to 'play' for a living and back that up with further research on the real power of play. Why is a play stage critical? Children learn through play. This is how our children explore the world around them and formulate ideas and higher-level concepts. Social play is, just as described, the basis for how our children engage in play with their peers. When we can clearly define where a child is performing, we can meet them in that stage, further expose them, and guide them through to the next stage. This also serves us as if you have been in a social setting with new mothers. It is a clear distinction that brings a sense of relief to a parent knowing that their 1-year-old prefers to play alone (and that this is age appropriate), as opposed to with his cousin, during the Thanksgiving gathering.

Before diving into Mildred Parten's research on the stages of play, I want to reframe the importance of 'play' as it relates to how a child learns. Let's think about the classic example of how most speech-language pathologists were taught academic skills needed for formal training on the job.

DOI: 10.4324/9781003491842-4

Our graduate school experience included all of the prerequisite courses as well as the clinical course work which were structured to provide us with the theoretical, anatomical, and clinical methods we would need to provide effective treatment and intervention in the field. However, our graduate course of study ended with a comprehensive examination, where, our skills just began to be 'put to the test' as we were given real-life 'case studies' to analyze and determine deficit from difference, assess and formulate a sound intervention plan. While the knowledge we gleaned from professors was invaluable, there was another portion which greatly tested our real understanding of the material, and that was clinical experience. I have to admit that the hands-on clinical aspect was paramount to learning and utilization of the methods that were taught in the classes of our graduate school. To switch this example back to the children we are training in specific skills, their 'hands on' learning is done through PLAY. They are testing their own hypotheses, watching how the world around them shifts as a result of certain behaviors, and so forth. As a result, I do believe that this chapter gleans a wealth of knowledge to speech-language pathologists, if nothing else but to help support the hard work that we do while "simply playing" with the children we serve.

Mildred Parten was a sociology professor who published a classic study that we still reference. It found distinct stages in play that guide a child's social progression as they grow and mature. Her research was based on observing preschool children, and she gleaned insight into how our children's social participation increased with age. Thus, Parten's social stages of play were born.

Unoccupied play is the first developmental stage in which a child merely explores their own body as it is in space; it is characterized as "a lot of random movements of arms and feet but no engagement with others." This stage typically does not appear to be play-based in nature but is merely a child occupying themselves by watching anything of passing interest. An example would be a 3-year-old who cannot sit and prefers to jump around the room, scanning for items to pick up and put in her mouth.

The second play stage is *onlooker play*, which is very much how it is labeled. It typically occurs after unoccupied play as it is the emergence of acknowledgment of others in their environment. This is when a child will observe others (mainly peers) but still need to engage with them. For many reasons, this supports social learning theory, suggesting that by observing others play more complexly, a child can pick up on those skills. At this stage, the child will typically ask questions, make suggestions, or bring items of interest to the playgroup, but not engage in play schemas.

Solitary play is generally the next sequential play stage in which a child is immersed in their toys. This is when children are so absorbed in their play that they often do not realize or care to engage with others around them. An example of solitary play would be engaging with Lego blocks since they work hard to improve their fine motor functions (e.g. building).

Parallel play is just as described; while children tend to play alone, they will play with similar toys to other children next to them. This is defined as a social stage because although they are not actively engaging with peers, they are playing with the same toys, making it social in nature.

Associative play is when there are loosely structured play activities in the group. Children will participate in an everyday activity (e.g. kitchen) but will have a different focus or goal. There are no real rules in associative play. However, it encourages children to get along with others and builds on language skills.

Cooperative play is when a child plays with a group with a group outcome. Examples of cooperative play include 'Simon Says' and role-playing play schemas.

While Mildred Parten was a sociology professor, she spoke about typical child play behavior; however, being speech-pathologists, we often see children who deviate from this norm, which is why we are hired to intervene. A classic example of a child who may not be hitting these stages would be a child who is three or four, still lining up cars in the corner of the room.

Common deficits would be a child who is on the autism spectrum. Children on the autism spectrum' defining characteristic is a lack of social engagement and interactions. This is pervasive beyond just peer play but extends to parents' interactions. We must also realize that social play requires background knowledge and exploration of a child's environment. The more complex stages (e.g. cooperative play – playing in the kitchen) require negotiating items in their environment, further language to navigate that environment, and knowledge of play schemas. If a child is primarily nonverbal and does not explore toys past banging them on the table, their social stage remains solitary until they gain core knowledge to support advancement.

Sample Milestone Score with Interventions/Case Study

The child is observed in the classroom; he watches his peers playing in the kitchen, every once in a while, walks over to the basket, takes out a play food item, and brings it to the children who are 'cooking with pans.' This child is in the associative play stage at the current moment. Their zone of intervention would be cooperative play. Intervention: Provide a direct model of taking those fruits and showing them to peers while providing an introductory example: "Doesn't the cake need some pineapple?" Incorporating questions (e.g. "Can Jonny and I have a turn to stir the sugar?"). Further active engagement with language models while interacting and facilitating the child's play in which you are serving.

Important Collaborative Considerations

When I speak about collaboration in relation to play skills I often think back to my ongoing work alongside various ABA (applied behavioral analysts) while working in the early intervention sector. While their training is highly structured, it does assist in shaping appropriate play for children who either can't or won't follow a social model. This can include the simple play task such as putting shapes in a sorter, completing a puzzle. I acknowledge that I am very broadly describing the work of an applied behavioral analysis (ABA) therapist, however, I have found them critical with my early intervention children who have a diagnosis of ASD (autism spectrum disorder), and working through a co-treatment model can really assist with functional play skills. Another professional who assists with such an area is an early childhood educator, even better if they have experience with SPED (the special education sector), as they utilize the same treatment strategies while intervening with children.

Preferred Methods and Procedures

There are various clinical and researched methods that assist with play-based interventions however, to name a few to reference which I personally align with: Floortime model, the Hanen Method (parent training based), and generally following the child's lead while they are exploring their environment.

The Floortime model (aka DIRFloortime) "is an approach used to promote an individual's development through a respectful, playful, joyful, and engaging process… it is based on the DIR model for human development." To be noted that this is a procedure in which clinicians are specifically trained in. The official website which provides a wealth of knowledge on Dr. Stanley Greenspan's work is cited below for further review (Greenspan, 2010).

An additional treatment source which I personally enjoy sharing with parents and educators is the Hanen Centre. The Hanen Approach is based on its key developer, Ayala Hanen Manolson; a speech-language pathologist out of Montreal, Canada who developed the program for groups of parents whose children had significant language delays. The main idea or takeaway from the Hanen approach is education and empowerment of parents to facilitate language learning and expression. Basically, empowering parents to be vital resources and 'teachers' for their child's language learning. The Hanen Centre has various programs for both parents and early childhood educators. I personally utilize their handouts to parents on my ClassDojo platforms as a method of monthly information for parents to 'digest' and ask follow-up questions on. For those of you who are not aware, ClassDojo is a remote platform in which therapists and teachers can connect with parents, both individually and as a group via messages and posts (*The Hanen Centre: Speech and language development for children*, 2016).

The model of generally 'getting on the child's level' is perhaps most visible when intervening in the preschool setting or in the homes (such as the early intervention program I touched on previously). The general 'gist' of the above mentioned in which I have gleaned is interact with whatever that child is interacting with AND model the more advanced skill. To begin, YOU (meaning the clinician), could be their 'peer' that they let into their play world. This can be as simple as utilizing a very simple bubble wand, where the clinician needs to blow the bubbles and the child needs to look at another and interact appropriately or request for more in a more collaborative model. The early concept of turn taking can additionally be introduced with such a simple toy, allowing the child to hold the wand and attempt to blow bubbles toward the clinician.

Mildred Parten (1932) Social stages of play

Stage of Development	Description	Age of Acquisition	Acquired (Y, N, Developing)
Solitary play	Play is solo; with their own ties. They don't typically get close to or interact with other children	Birth –2 years	
Onlooker play	Child watching but not making attempt to join	Birth +	
Parallel play	Play is still solo but often next to (or parallel) to others	2.5–3.5 years	
Associative play	Begin to play with others by sharing toys (still may have their own play-line)	3–4.5 years	

(Continued)

(Continued)

Stage of Development	Description	Age of Acquisition	Acquired (Y, N, Developing)
Cooperative play	Children play in groups cooperatively to achieve common goal. Requires negotiation (where children can change roles/take turns and accept suggestions about play)	4–5.5 years	
Games with rules	Cooperative play that includes winners and losers. Children make the rules to these games (not like competitive sports). Demonstrate understanding of social rules in culture.	6+ years	

References

Drew, C., & Cornell, D. (2023, October 11). *Parten's 6 stages of play in childhood, explained!* Helpful Professor. https://helpfulprofessor.com/stages-of-play/

Greenspan, S. (2010). *What is floortime?* Home of DIRFloortime® (Floortime). https://www.icdl.com/floortime

The Hanen Centre | Speech and Language Development for Children. (2016). *The Hanen Centre: Speech and language development for children.* https://www.hanen.org/Home.aspx

5 Cognitive Milestones

Cognitive milestones can glean some insight into a child's general functioning. These milestones allow us to form a basis for how the child explores their world and interacts with their environment, and general milestones to identify if their current functioning is within normal bounds. I also find that certain milestones (e.g. can label colors) are helpful for speech-pathologists as we can also target specific areas in our intervention. Knowledge of cognitive milestones makes a holistic intervention all-encompassing, with collaboration between disciplines and targets. In other words, instead of the speech therapist standing alone in interventions, collaboration and cross-referencing other areas can assist in multiple opportunities for cross-discipline interventions. In particular, regarding pre-academic skills, cognitive functioning milestones can assist us when coaching parents and young educators. In particular, concerning attention to task, did you know that an average 5-year-old can attend between 5 and 10 minutes at any given time? Information on attention span is paramount and can assist with distinguishing between a difference and a disorder when we see kindergarteners outside these norms.

I like to think of cognitive milestones as the process where a young child's brain is wiring itself to make connections between himself and the outside world. A clear example would be a typical 4-month-old putting items in their mouth to explore them; you expect this for a young child, however, a 4-year-old who mouths everything as a means to explore is performing lower in the cognitive functioning skill area. How does knowledge in these milestones assist us in therapy? It reminds us to what extent to 'meet a child where they are functioning' instead of coming at them with higher-level expectations (e.g. sitting and reading a book to a child who is mouthing everything as a means to explore).

I have formulated the below-mentioned cognitive milestones from the most readily available list available, that of the United States Center for Disease Control (CDC). What I found particularly interesting about the milestones are their correlation and integration of various other areas of

DOI: 10.4324/9781003491842-5

development, namely speech and language related. They span from social and relational milestones (e.g. "watches caregiver as they move") to the more complex (e.g. "writes some letters in their name"). There is an interconnectedness between the cognitive milestones and other milestones such as Piaget's sensorimotor stage which addresses the concept of object permanence (cognitive milestone, as it's listed below "looks for toys/preferred items that are out of sight"). I especially found this informational chart to be helpful as it is in correlation with the other areas of The Protocol, and therefore, goals that are gleaned from one area of The Protocol can supplement goals in another 'area.'

Related Case Studies

Case Study 1

Alice
3-year-old/female
Alice is a 3-year-old attending preschool who has been in school for about 12 months now. Alice enjoys banging toys on the table and grabbing desired toys to mouth them as a means of exploration. She does not yet have object permanence, so when you take the binky out of her mouth and put it out of direct sight she will throw herself on the floor. Alice will not put items in a container (e.g. putting rattle in the box when music is over). Her mother states that everything goes in her mouth and she does not seem to interact in any meaningful way.

Alice's current level of functioning: "Exploring items with mouth"

Alice's area of intervention: Object permanence and putting items in a container.

Object permanence permits our children to learn that just because objects are out of sight does not mean that they have ceased to exist all together. This also can glean insight into the rationale behind why children have serious separation anxiety. Let's think about it, if you thought that every time your family member walked out of the room that you would never see them again how would you feel?

Treatment: With Alice, I used a toy known as the 'what's inside box' and put items in a clear box with a blanket over the top. Successive approximation to assist the student in finding items in the box, a further demonstration of putting items IN box with hand-over-hand demonstration. This activity is done while using basic noises during interactions (e.g. "oops, uh oh, mmm"). This is where a slightly sheer cloth placed over a favored toy can assist in demonstrating this concept of object permanence.

To address the second milestone of putting items together in play or interaction, I like to introduce this during routines with a child so they feel safe and comfortable exploring toys and stimuli in a new way. I like to use the opportunity during classroom transition time to sing a song (cue 'clean up song') and help them via hand over hand to take toys and put them in the box. Additionally, I recommend Alice's mom take the towel after her bath is done and drop it into the laundry bag. A child in this stage will generally like the cause and effect of certain items (name the laundry bag with a top) and Mom can incorporate open/shut while Alice is exploring the laundry bag.

Case Study 2

Johnny

3 years 5 months, male

Johnny, another preschooler, loves to collect all of the toys in the classroom and line them up. Does this sound familiar? He will look for favored items the teachers often hide (e.g. miniature moose) and will pretend to sweep the floor in the classroom when the teachers sing the clean up song.

Johnny's current level of functioning: Copies chores and routine tasks and plays with objects in simple ways.

Johnny's area of intervention: Play with more than one toy at a time, pretend play.

Treatment: While Johnny loves to use the swiffer when the teacher tells the children to clean up, he will often leave the dust in a pile despite being shown the dustbin and the garbage. I utilized Johnny's love of the swiffer to expand upon his use of one object to two objects together. I helped him after he was done sweeping to push the dust into the bin, and then; using two hands dump it in the garbage can. To build on his interest in miniature animals, I introduced the pretend play paddock with plastic food and demonstrated taking turns feeding the zebra and other animals. At this point, I utilized narration of actions he made with the zebra ("oh zebra walking!") as well as my own ("my moose is hungry! Can he have some hay?,"- pointing to the hay next to Johnny's zebra).

Case Study 3

Nina

4.5-year-old/female

Nina was a climber who also happens to love plastic bags, so much so that the teachers needed to leave the trash can outside of the classroom because of the fits which ensued after she was denied free access. Nina, to my surprise, would see a bag on the counter of the speech room and commence jumping on top of the nearest chair to grab that plastic bag. Believe it or not, this is a basic problem-solving skill. The beloved plastic bag is on top of the counter and I need it. She even answered the 'how' question herself.

Nina's current level of functioning: Demonstrates simple problem-solving skills

Nina's area of intervention: Follows two-step directions

Treatment: I knew that motivation was extremely high for Nina to get to her beloved plastic bag, which fed itself into the two-step direction task. While we started with preferred items as motivators (namely the bag), I demonstrated simple first/then language with associated visuals (e.g. first, shoes and socks on, then come to the door and wait to go to the speech room (showing her the item of preference)). While this is a conditional two-step direction, it eventually became routine and I was able to increase motivation and engagement based on time spent with Nina's preferred stimuli.

Important Collaborative Measures

Regarding cognitive milestones, most of our older children (preschool and up) have a more comprehensive psychological battery of tests. These tests often include the following for your reference: Wechsler Preschool and Primary Scale of Intelligence (WPPSI), Wechsler Intelligence Scale for Children (WISC), Differential Ability Scales (DAS), Stanford-Binet, among others. These tests dive into a vast array of cognitive functioning, including verbal comprehension, visual and spatial skills, fluid reasoning, working memory, and processing speed. Regarding cognitive development, this is an area where collaboration with the psychologist is paramount, as we can glean information behind where a child is functioning cognitively to cater speech interventions accordingly. To be noted, while this text is geared toward speech-language pathologists who are primarily treating the pediatric population, speech-language pathologists do utilize assessments and screeners to sample an adult's cognitive functioning. To provide a comprehensive overview, I have screeners which I have utilized and collaborated with treating physicians in the subacute sector as long as long-term care which include Mini-mental State Examination (MMSE), the Montreal Cognitive Assessment (MoCA), and the Saint Louis University Mental Status Examination (SLUMS). All of the above-mentioned adult screeners can be utilized with the population of 15 years and up, with allowances made for those who are illiterate (as there is a written component) as well as academic schooling considerations. The above-mentioned tests which can be performed on adults are just touching the tip of the iceberg of the cognitive interventions that we can perform as speech-language pathologists. The purpose in mentioning them is to empower speech-pathologists to enter the discussion during academic meetings regarding a child's cognition and functioning, as certain cognitive abilities (e.g. memory) can be facilitated through our interventions.

Preferred Methods and Procedures

Again, this is an area where meeting the child where they are currently functioning is vital. When we are able to get into their current level of functioning (no matter what it is), we are able to assist in bridging that gap between where they are and a more advanced developmental stage. To support this, more of a child-directed approach can greatly assist with children who have cognitive deficits. To add to the recommendation, a child who is not functioning in an age-appropriate way, cognitively benefits from assistance with activities of daily living (or ADL's). Intervention is best performed while they are going about their daily activities. This is for two reasons, we learn through repetition of a task, and with an activity or task that is completed every day and/or multiple times a day, their repetition and exposure are increased. The second reason for utilization of everyday activities to teach basic cognitive skills is their parents and family will be involved in these tasks and can perform, under our direction, as a vital facilitator in teaching the belowmentioned skills.

Milestone	Typical Age of Acquisition	Acquired (All, Some)
Watches caregiver as they move	2 months	
Looks at toy for several seconds	2 months	
Opens mouth for bottle if hungry	4 months	
Looks at own hands with interest	4 months	
Puts items in mouth to explore them	4 months	
Reaches to grab at desired toys	4 months	
Will demonstrate he's done with food by closing mouth	4 months	
Looks for toys/preferred items that are out of sight (object permanence)	9 months	
Bangs two items together	9 months	
Puts items in a container (e.g. block in a cup)	12 months	
Looks for items he sees you hide (e.g. stuffy under a blanket)	12 months	
Interacts with items the right way (demonstrates functional knowledge of items) (e.g. tries to talk on phone, will know to eat banana)	15 months	
Will stack at least two items (e.g. two blocks)	15 months	
Copies chores or routine activities (e.g. sweeping the floor, cleaning the dishes)	18 months	
Plays in toys in simple ways (e.g. pushing car)	18 months	

(*Continued*)

(Continued)

Milestone	Typical Age of Acquisition	Acquired (All, Some)
Can hold one item in one hand while simultaneously using the other hand to do something else (e.g. holding a cup and pouring with a teacup with the other hand)	2 years	
Attempts to use switches, knobs, zippers on toys	2 years	
Plays with more than one toy at a time (e.g. can take food out of play microwave and put it on a plate)	2 years	
Begins pretend play (e.g. feeding baby doll)	30 months	
Demonstrates simple problem solving skills (e.g. stands on stool to reach counter)	30 months	
Follows two-step directions (e.g. get your shoes and bring them to the door)	30 months	
Knows at least one color (e.g. show me blue)	30 months	
Can draw a circle with direct model	3 years	
Avoids touching hot stove when given warning (safety awareness)	3 years	
Can label a number of colors	4 years	
Basic sequencing skills (can tell you what happens next in a familiar storybook)	4 years	
Draws a person with 3+ body parts	4 years	
Counts to 10	5 years	
Can label some colors when pointed to (from 1 to 5)	5 years	
Demonstrates understanding of time by using temporal words (e.g. yesterday, tomorrow, today)	5 years	
Can attend for 5–10 minutes on one task	5 years	
Writes some letters in their name	5 years	
Can name some letters when pointed to	5 years	

Level of mastery
Zone of intervention
Age expectation

Reference

CDC's Developmental Milestones. (2022, 17 August). *Centers for disease control and prevention.*Centers for Disease Control and Prevention. https://www.cdc.gov/ncbddd/actearly/milestones/index.html

6 Receptive Language Milestones

Receptive language, in layperson's terms, is arguably the building block of language as we know it. To appropriately and actively engage in our environment, we need first to understand the language in which we are immersed. How I describe this language portion to families and teachers is what their child understands OR the directions their child follows. As a major building block of language as we know it, receptive language can arguably be the first area to begin intervention, as we need labels and meaning behind the language to understand the world around us. As you may notice, the earlier receptive milestones are all related to response to the environment. This is another reason why we are encouraged to double-check a child's audiogram or hearing to ensure they hear their environmental stimuli. For quick reference, an audiogram is a measurement that audiologists utilize to test an individual's hearing acuity. More of the nuanced receptive language milestones, such as tone of voice and general attention and tracking, are listed in these very first months. While it may be tempting for us to pass over this portion of language when assessing and intervening with their speech, these milestones can be paramount when working with children who have not even reached a state of joint attention and engagement with caregivers. Joint attention being: "when one person purposefully coordinates their focus of attention with that of another person" (*About joint attention*, n.d.). For example, as you may notice, a typically developing child between 4 and 6 months of age enjoys songs and music. This tidbit of developmental preference can greatly guide intervention both on the 1:1 sessions and recommendations for carryover at home. Let me provide an example: I have had a whole slew of children who love songs. While they may not yet have the attention span to sit for a book or complete a simple puzzle, they will happily bob along to the wheels on the bus, for instance. This is our entryway into skilled and guided intervention for receptive language. Take a child where they are functioning (e.g. loves music and songs) and use this to develop their receptive language further, e.g. provide two items (wheels, wipers) and ask the child to 'take wheels' with associated movement.

DOI: 10.4324/9781003491842-6

Deficits in receptive language would be described as a baby not engaging in their environment, not turning their head toward noise, or tracking it. This could also present as a child who does not respond to their parents when they call their name. As an older child, receptive language deficits can present themselves in difficulty following complex directions in the classroom. This can look like the child who is still playing in the corner while the rest of the children are getting packed up and ready for lunch. A more subtle receptive language deficit could look like the child who is constantly looking to their peers in the classroom for the next step or activity, requiring their models to identify what is being asked of them.

Generally, receptive language can be linked with comprehension deficits. Language is not tangible at first. We learn vocabulary and language through our interactions with these items in our natural environment. This is where the level of cognitive functioning comes into play. As we learn that an actual car is most accessible to identify, a miniature item is second, moving on to a colored photograph. Such receptive language deficits can be correlated with cognitive deficits, intellectual disabilities, or even a child who is on the autism spectrum and is entirely self-directed and unable to attend for long enough to learn the vocabulary for said favorite toy.

Related Case Studies with Sample Milestone Score with Interventions

Alan
3 years 2 months
Alan absolutely loves books that have animals. He would saunter into the speech room and stare at the bookcase, all while wringing his hands and making stimulatory sounds while scanning for a book that is of interest. As far as functional speech, Alan would imitate non-speech sounds such as "beep" and makes an approximation of the lip blueberry sound when he saw elephants. Any time I would make the elephant noise he would stop what he was doing and look at my lips intently.

Current Milestone: Imitates non-speech sounds (infrequently)
Area of intervention: Identifies pictures
Alan was a stickler for routine. Which means that he loved it when I got out my song books during therapy sessions. I utilized the associated songbook (e.g. Old McDonald) and sing-along to ask what the cow says. Alan made an approximation of 'moo' at which point I said "yes." While he knew the associated sound with the familiar object I asked him to 'show me what animal says 'moo!' While Alan originally wanted me to make all the animal noises at once without waiting for my direction or instruction, I was able to shape his understanding of the noise (an area in which he excelled in) with the label of the animal. After which Alan was able to 'point to' elephant!'

The method utilized the current milestone the child had mastered to target the next developmental skill. Since the associated stimuli are preferred or familiar based on the noise it makes, it can bridge the gap between non-identification and accurate identification.

Shane
3 years 1 month
Shane loved the Cocomelon bathtub toy that was a permanent fixture in the speech therapy room, he also loved the associated songs the toy echoed from its speakers. Besides being overly interested in noisy toys, Shane was able to understand the meaning of 'no' as he would stop what he was doing when he heard this word. Shane did not, however, respond to his name consistently when called.

Current milestone/s: Responds to name and no.

Area of intervention: Enjoys and attempts to engage in games (e.g. pattycake)

During speech sessions, I would be saying "Shane" more than half the sessions. I encouraged him to respond to his name by acknowledging when he turned his head (e.g. "Shane!" child turns head, "Shane, want to play peek-a-boo?"). I was able to engage Shane in a simple peek-a-boo with a dolly and wash cloth/blankie, utilizing his name and waiting for him to fill in the blank in a familiar routine. "Peek- a-... Expectant pause" "boo" "Peek a boo, Shane!"

This utilizes his current mastery level of responding to his name and works in his targeted engagement area in simple games.

Rachel
2 years 5 months
Rachel was a ball of energy who adored everything related to nursery rhymes and songs. She would often be spotted dancing down the hall when a coworker forgot to shut off their ringtone. While Rachel was able to point to pictures of favored stimuli (e.g. Peppa pig show), was able to grab a maraca out of the teacher's hand to shake it during circle time, and label basic items around the classroom (namely her backpack), she was unable to label anything more than her 'eyes.'

Current milestone: Points to pictures in a book, once named. Follow 1-step direction (put maraca in box).

Area of intervention: Labels a few body parts and understands simple stories.

Rachel enjoyed everything related to a game, which I used in my favor. This is where I re-introduced "Head, shoulders, knees and toes" song. Once we had run through it, after first providing hand-over-hand support so she could "get it" I would utilize expectant pause for Rachel to fill in the blank "head..." with a gesture to the shoulder. I obviously took approximations at this time as we were not working on articulation but rather body part identification. I then added more body parts into the game and even turned this into a game with another student in the room where Rachel and he would play a version of Simon Says. Relating to stories, I had exactly the book I was going to pull from my arsenal to play Rachel, one which had great rhythm and rhyme; I grabbed "Pete the Cat and his new shoes" and before long Rachel was learning the sequencing of the story and was singing along with the refrain of the book.

Important Collaborative Measures

Due to the importance of receptive language and its impact on everyday lives and pre-academic skills, this is a critical time to ensure that the necessary referrals are made. If a child is not responding to their name at 12 months of age, refer them to an audiologist. I would like to take this opportunity to bring up the topic of potential hearing loss and how a hearing screener and follow-up test is crucial from a very young age. As mentioned previously, many of the earliest of receptive language milestones are based on tracking sounds and others in their environment, if a child is not hearing appropriately these milestones are automatically not being met. Therefore, as a general rule of thumb, it is critical for us to request hearing screening results that are up to date for children when we are first referred for a child's speech and language development. We can also request this for adults that come into our practice as well, as the inability to respond to questions appropriately can be due to a hearing loss as opposed to a receptive language deficit. In my years of working as a speech-language pathologist I have had more adult clients who had hearing loss than children, however, in the cases in which I have had children with sensorineural hearing loss, outfitting of hearing aides and various other devices has been CRUCIAL in receptive and expressive language development. How can you learn appropriately when you cannot hear? In upcoming chapters, I will discuss more in-depth speech sound frequencies and reference the hearing acuity needed for an individual to hear certain sounds so bookmark this for later reference. For the purposes of this chapter, ensure that your clients have passed a hearing screening by an audiologist and/or a full hearing test. Ensure the child has a full workup regarding hearing to rule out any deficits. If the child is not able to actively track the parents' voice, a potential developmental pediatrician referral or educational specialist may be in line to rule out any underlying issues or comorbidities.

Preferred Methods and Procedures

As I am sure you will notice, the receptive language milestones ceiling out at 4 years of age on the belowmentioned chart, however, they are the foundation to higher-level receptive language skills. Additionally, since these foundational receptive language skills are based on hearing stimuli in their environment, I utilize loud or noisy toys to gain and further sustain attention with my little ones. I will cycle out toys, meaning there is only one noisy toy in the environment at a time, to not overwhelm a child auditorily. If a child's joint attention is deemed appropriate, I will alternatively take out the batteries of basic toys such as an animal puzzle that usually has a button to make the noise itself, in order to stimulate expressive language skills (e.g. child making the noise of a sheep, or my imitation of the noise). The emphasis of exaggerated intonation and speech in the early months is paramount and I utilize various inflections while providing speech and language intervention through the early months of intervention with children. If you are curious as to what this looks or sounds like, Google Miss Rachel on YouTube. I have not dived into her credentials, however, MANY of the strategies she utilizes on her online platform are utilized by speech-language pathologists for years; I believe this is the reason for her wild success and accessibility to parents and educators.

To name a few of the strategies that assist in receptive language growth with the youngest of children: expectant pause, emphasis on certain labels or names at a slow rate, exclamations, exaggeration of facial expressions and associated gestures. I often utilize basic baby signs along with directions provided to my younger babies (e.g. /stop/ sign with the 'no' directive), I will often make an exclamation to associate with such a direction such as 'ouch!' when I am pointing to an object that could be harmful (e.g. scissor or sharp table corner). Receptive language, or language understanding, is learned through hands-on experience, therefore often physical prompts assist in teaching skills such as 'put the block IN the box' (with associated clean-up song); therefore, when teaching the earlier receptive language skills maximal verbal, visual, and tactile cues are often employed to assist in growing our children's neuronal connections and language understanding.

I often utilize the belowmentioned milestones IN my intervention. For example, a child of 4 to 6 months "enjoys music and rhythm." This is where I have printed and laminated nursery song folders to engage them in daily songs at the beginning of therapy sessions. The receptive language portion of /Five little Speckled Frogs/? Was the direction of 'take frog' as the frogs are 'jumping' into the water and off the folder. Therapy materials which have rhythm and rhyme as well as repetition are helpful with the development of both receptive and expressive languages as they are easy for a child to memorize and become familiar with. This is where receptive and expressive languages intersect in our children's early years and this works wonderfully for our therapy!

Yet another example of particularly engaging activities to conduct with our young children, as it relates to receptive language skills, are songs related to skills they should acquire at such an age. Such a song /Head, Shoulders, Knees, and Toes/ can target the 'point to a few body parts' milestone which is expected around 12 months of age.

Again, I will fall back on the importance of embedding language and learning IN everyday activities and hands-on experiences. There is an opportunity for receptive language learning ANYWHERE a child is and, an innumerable amount of toys, will *not* serve us if we do not engage appropriately with children to teach the belowmentioned skills. I have found it best to utilize some toys a child has in their own home, or pull out my song folders to demonstrate to parents just how we can grow our children's understanding of language by the way we interact with their environment – not the added 'noise' or toys that often are added to the storage boxes in the corner of our family's living room.

Milestone	Age of Mastery	Acquired (Yes, No, Approaching/ Scattered)
Startle or cry to unexpected noise	Birth	
Wake up to loud noises	Birth	
Stop moving upon hearing new and unfamiliar noises	Birth	
Turn head toward caregivers voice	3 months	
Smile when hear parents voice	3 months	
Stop what they are doing and listen closely to a new noise	0–3 months	
Respond to comforting tone of voice (familiar or not)	0–3 months	
Respond to "no"	4–6 months	
Respond to different tones of voice	4–6 months	
Responds to noises other than talking (e.g. car driving by)	4–6 months	
Attends to toys and objects that make noise	4–6 months	
Enjoy music and rhythm	4–6 months	
Responds to their name (by turning and looking at the person calling them)	7–12 months	
Enjoys and attempts to participate in simple games (e.g. patty cake)	7–12 months	
Recognize the name of familiar objects (e.g. car, cookie, shoe)	7–12 months	
Imitates non-speech sounds (e.g. animal sounds "moo" "beep")	9–12 months	
Identifies pictures	12–15 months	
Displays object use (e.g. knows what to do with a cup, ball)	12–15 months	
Follows one-step directions	21–24 months	
Points to pictures in a book once named	1–2 years	

(*Continued*)

(Continued)

Milestone	Age of Mastery	Acquired (Yes, No, Approaching/ Scattered)
Can point to a few body parts (e.g. nose, mouth, ear)	1–2 years	
Follows simple commands (e.g. "push the car")	1–2 years	
Understands simple questions (e.g. "where's the car?")	1–2 years	
Listens to simple stories	1–2 years	
Enjoys songs and rhymes	1–2 years	
Enjoys repetition of favored stories/songs and rhymes	1–2 years	
Identifies clothing items and their pictures	18–21 months	
Understands "come here" direction	18–21 months	
Uses two-word phrases	18–21 months	
Understands two-step directions (e.g. "get your shirt and put it in the hamper")	2–3 years	
Understands contrasting concepts (e.g. big/small, hot/cold)	2–3 years	
Recognized doorbell ringing or phone (demonstrated by pointing and showing excitement)	2–3 years	
Understands simple "who" "where" and "what" questions	2–3 years	
Can hear you and come when you call from another room (out of sight)	2–3 years	
Can answer simple 'wh' questions about stories	3–4 years	
Demonstrates understanding of the conversations going on at home, daycare etc.	3–4 years	

(Bowen, 1998).

Level of mastery
Zone of intervention
Age expectation

References

Bowen, C. (1998). Typical speech and language acquisition in infants and young children. https://www.speech-language-therapy.com/

UNC School of Medicine. (n.d.). *About joint attention*. https://www.med.unc.edu/healthsciences/asap/materials-1/about-joint-attention/

7   Expressive Language Milestones

Expressive language is what parents and colleagues ask us about when it comes to a child's language development. This is perhaps because expressive language is the most outward demonstration of our children's understanding of language and the world around them. If I am being sincere, it is the main reason why I was drawn into the field of speech pathology, the desire to give others 'their voice.' What I particularly loved when researching the steps and evidence of a child's expressive language development is the incorporation of multi-modes to express like, dislike, needs, and wants. These milestones can also support and encourage caregivers, as an essential smile or even vocal play has communicative intent and meaning from the early age of 0 to 3 months of age. In particular, this area can assist us in identifying successive ways to intervene and shape a child's expressive language to approximate more natural and functional communication. While this section of The Protocol dives into expressive language at an early age, we can think back on how we (as adults) express ourselves. It could be through writing or singing, through hobbies. Either way, it is essential for our daily functioning to have the means to express our thoughts and feelings. As you will see, expressive language milestones (e.g. labels six body parts) correlate with receptive language milestones (e.g. can identify six body parts), assisting us in skilled intervention targets while planning daily and weekly sessions with our clients.

I would like to use this time to note that expressive language does not have to be verbal. This often is received as a shock from most parents and colleagues, as in: "my daughter received a point on testing because she merely pointed to what she wanted?" or "this entails my son throwing himself on the ground because he doesn't want to do something?" This is the domain under which nonverbal communication would fall under. Think about it, if you do not have the words to express desires, wants, hopes, what would you resort to in order to have your needs known? Most likely whatever means that are available to you and, after working with children for over a decade, I can say this often manifests itself

DOI: 10.4324/9781003491842-7

into tantrums and physical reactions. This is the area where methodology and training in more 'functional communication' is paramount! Whether the functional communication be basic baby signs (e.g. all done, more), gestures (e.g. shaking head), or even the utilization of an augmentative alternative communication (AAC) device, all are methods to bridge the gap between a non-functional communicator and a proficient one.

When I think about expressive language acquisition, I am brought immediately back to a summer internship at a preschool autistic classroom. I was, like other undergraduates, unaware of what I wanted to do with my Bachelor of Arts in Psychology degree upon college graduation (which was two years away) when my father recommended I work as an aide for the summer program. I was assigned as a personal aide to a little girl with Rett's disorder. I will call her Ally. Ally had beautiful ringlets which her mother tastefully would put up in a half ponytail. Ally had the wide, unsteady gait that most Rett's children have and was primarily nonverbal. She did make what I can describe as self-stimulatory noises (e.g. ahhh) while she would rock back and forth and wring her hands in the classroom. There were many times when Ally would become frustrated and fling herself onto the ground or cry as a means to communicate. This was when I met the speech-pathologist, who utilized a binary touch chat at the time to assist in basic functional requests. In Ally's case, the AAC device (augmentative alternative communication) served as her method to successfully communicate to her parents and school staff. The AAC device was Ally's 'voice.'

At the start of the summer program, there were at least 10 out of the 12 children who were exhibiting aversive behaviors (e.g. screaming, tantrums, etc.). By the time the program ended these same children had acquired functional communication. I recall the very first word that a little 5-year-old uttered during lunchtime. I grew to love my time as an aide in that summer program. To provide a child a 'voice,' to assist in making their daily life that much easier, to help them feel understood, this, I thought, would be a "job" that would not feel like work.

To this day I have worked with clients of all ages from 3 months to 104 years old, and I can still say that providing my clients with a means to express themselves is the "gift that keeps giving" me a deep sense of satisfaction.

Causes of Deficiencies

Deficits in expressive language are the most apparent to people outside of our field. This can look like a child making high-pitched screams at 3½ years old without actual words or meaning. It can be as simple as a child with a limited vocabulary (e.g. four words – cookie, mommy, daddy, doggie) at the age of 2. It can also manifest itself in the middle of the grocery store when you observe a child screaming inconsolably in the aisle without using a purposeful point or gesture to demonstrate his needs or wants.

This area's deficiencies can be due to a lack of exposure to the outside world, inconsistent language models, learning deficits, or neurological deficits. This is where I commonly tell parents of young children to 'label everything!' A label is one word; accompany it with a point, and you have a multi-modal form of communication on your hands.

While our work with the pediatric population exhibits expressive language deficits which are a combination of nature and nurture responses, expressive language deficits with the adult population can result from more neurological incidents. Neurological incidents which I will mention here, as a means to be comprehensive, include dementia, Parkinson's disease, cerebrovascular incidents (CVA's), transient ischemic attack (TIA), traumatic brain injury (TBI) to name a few. To be noted, working with the older pediatric population (e.g. children over 14 years of age) can yield deficits resulting from TBI's, especially if they are engaged in hands-on sports which can cause brain injury or damage.

Related Case Studies with Sample Milestone Score and Interventions

Case Study 1

Anna "loves songs" and will turn her head and babble in response; she does not yet imitate non-speech sounds (e.g. "beep.")

Skilled Intervention

1 Introduce 'wheels on the bus' with the use of expectant pause, over articulation, and slowing rate of speech model while engaging in the song.
2 Use of manipulatives to accompany parts (e.g. wheels).
3 Shape this to further labels of buses and vehicles on the street while Mom takes her out in the stroller.

Case Study 2

Jacob laughs and produces 'b' and raspberries with his mouth. He likes to bounce around in his pack-and-play. He does not yet babble!

Skilled intervention: Practice assisting with bouncing with emphasis on basic CV combinations; 'up!' 'maa- for more.' Utilize expectant pauses while engaging the child in movement (which he prefers) to target the next sequential intervention area.

Important Collaborative Measures

Expressive language is a speech-language pathologist's niche – most of us thrive in teaching and expanding our children's communicative repertoire, making us experts. However, there are times when collaboration is necessary, such as for multilingual children with hearing loss or other physiological issues (e.g. breathing), in which referrals should be made to a bilingual therapist, audiologist, and respiratory therapist. Some children additionally have difficulty with sequencing and timing mechanisms, indicating potential childhood apraxia of speech (CAS). This is where a skilled and succinct multimodal strategy, such as prompt-trained therapy, comes into important play. I would be remiss if I omitted the potential of augmentative alternative communication (AAC) collaboration for children who cannot even engage in vocal play during interactions.

Methods and Procedures

To refer back to treatment strategies which were briefly addressed in the introductory chapter, this is where methods such as expectant pause, fill-in-the-blanks, exaggerated intonation, as well as language modeling and recasting are all strategies which are paramount in developing and expanding a child's expressive language abilities. Expressive language is interactional in nature, our 'voice' is the vehicle which shares our thoughts and ideas with the world around us; therefore, we teach these skills by modeling them ourselves.

To provide some examples for context, a child who is babbling during mealtime will often respond when you 'mimic' or mirror the sounds they are utilizing while adding appropriate speech sound productions. Let's say a child is saying 'nanana' while chewing on a soft spoon in the presence of the therapist and mother; this can easily be shaped into a 'mamama' mmmmm'! Sound and sound combination is appropriate to the context (eating food that is 'mmm' yummy!). From a cognitive development perspective, labels and verbal approximations are easier to identify for a child if they are IN their environment – meaning an actual banana is easier to identify than a photo of a banana, they will make the correlation between the label of the item and the production of that label ('nana').

I additionally like to pull out the "help me" or "I don't know" trick with my younger children who I want to 'label' objects they want. I will do this by looking where they are pointing and purposefully grabbing an item next to the item they desire, requiring them to correct me. This is where a mand model is utilized. For those of you who are not aware of what 'mand model' is, it is when a clinician will withhold an item that is desired until the child gives the appropriate request (or verbal approximation of the label) before giving it to them. When the child corrects me with an appropriate verbal approximation (e.g., "bana" for "banana"), I will repeat, "Oh, BANANA" slowly. Then I'll say, "Silly Stephy, did you mean 'banana'?" while handing them the item. This way, I can prompt another verbal approximation, helping them use functional labels to request their preferred items.

Another method that I like to utilize when we are touching on expressive language development is the utilization of binary choice. In referring to the below-mentioned chart 'asks for more' during mealtime, I will often stop and ask the child 'more' or 'all done'? With associated baby signs. Eventually the children will drop the sign and approximate 'ma' for more in which turn they will get 'more' of the desired food. Notice how we are not only targeting expressive language labels, BUT we are addressing receptive language targets as well (the concepts of more and all done or finished).

The expressive language milestones that are listed below are directly from not only ASHA but Caroline Bowen who additionally updates the stages as necessary.

Milestone	Age of Mastery	Acquired? Yes, No, Some?
Make different sounds for pleasure or pain	0–3 months	
Smiles upon seeing caregiver	0–3 months	
Coo's or goo's or makes same sound when happy	0–3 months	
Produces different cries for different reasons (e.g. pain, hungry)	0–3 months	
Turns head to voices	3–6 months	
Babbles and laughs	3–6 months	
Produces /b, p, m/ consonants	3–6 months	
Gurgling or vocal play when entertained	4–6 months	
Begin babbling (begins with bilabials /p, b, w, m/)	4–6 months	
Uses sounds and gestures to indicate what they want	4–6 months	
Attends to pictures	6–9 months	
Attends to singing	6–9 months	
Responds to sounds of things he/she can't see	6–9 months	

(*Continued*)

(Continued)

Milestone	Age of Mastery	Acquired? Yes, No, Some?
More advanced babbling (new consonants and CV combinations with both long and short vowels)	7–12 months	
Uses speech or other sounds (other than crying) to get parents attention and communicate needs	7–12 months	
Imitates non-speech sounds (e.g. animal sounds "moo" "beep")	9–12 months	
First words or first word approximations! (e.g. "mama, night night")	7–12 months	
Shakes head "no"	12–15 months	
Names objects (e.g. ball, cup, milk)	12–15 months	
Labels 6 body parts	15–18 months	
Asks for "more"	15–18 months	
Verbalizes for various reasons (e.g. wants, needs, emotions)	18–21 months	
Uses 50–100 words	21–24 months	
Uses plurals	21–24 months	

Level of mastery

Zone of intervention
Age expectation

Reference

Bowen, C. (1998). Typical speech and language acquisition in infants and young children. https://www.speech-language-therapy.com/

8 Motor Speech Progressions

Motor speech is the programming and timing of the coarticulation of words, phrases, and eventual sentences and paragraphs. I like to describe motor speech as the analogy of: you cannot run until you walk or walk before you can crawl, etc. It stands on the basis that we need a strong foundation before advancing to more complex concepts. The same is true for the coarticulation of speech. For example, if a baby isn't making vowel sounds (e.g. ahh, ooo) while riding in the carriage or being bounced on mama's lap, how will they progress to words like banana or speaking in full sentences? In particular, motor speech and deficits in this area can escalate to potential apraxia of speech. For children, this is known as childhood apraxia of speech. This translates to the deficit in motor timing and programming of the articulators during speech sound production. A child with childhood apraxia of speech (CAS) will often exhibit groping during attempted label and multisyllabic word production. They will not produce consistent words or word combinations and appear disorganized with their speech sound production and coarticulation. This is where a motor programming complexity chart can come in handy, guiding speech therapists toward areas of concern and targets.

Causes of Deficiencies

Deficits in motor speech include a child making all open-mouth vowel noises without any consonants in their repertoire. An example of a motor speech deficit is a child making animal noises (e.g. moo, woo) but without clear labels. Additionally, this can look like a child who makes inconsistent errors – with spare instances where he/she produces a word correctly. Since speech requires highly specialized motor programming to map out the appropriate coarticulatory production of words there are many reasons why a child could be unable to progress as his typical peers. A child with a developmental delay, cleft lip or palate, Down's syndrome, or cranial

DOI: 10.4324/9781003491842-8

nerve damage can exhibit difficulties with coarticulation. A childhood acquired disorder could include the example of Moebius syndrome, which I have mentioned previously in my introductory chapter. This is an acquired disorder in which the facial nerve is damaged either during or shortly after birth. Due to the fact that the facial nerve innervates with other valuable cranial nerves for speech sound production and coarticulation, difficulty with speech programming and timing occurs.

Motor speech can additionally encompass a larger range of deficits that can impact both our pediatric and adult populations. Dysarthric speech can be acquired at a young age as well, as I had a child in my time of practice who was of the middle school age and had speech which was dysarthric in nature. As a refresher, dysarthric speech often results in slow and slurred production. This can be caused by damage to the brain. My speech-language pathologist colleagues who have hands-on experience working with the geriatric and adult populations would attest to the prevalence of this motor speech deficit as well.

When we are talking about motor speech, there needs to be discussion around the oral motor mechanism and evaluation of the speech sound structures (e.g. lingual, labial, and dentition). This is why an oral motor examination (aka OME) WITH a diadochokinetic rate test is paramount. The diadochokinesis (DDK) does glean information regarding a child's coarticulation, motor programming, and timing, and it is easy to conduct. Therefore, common causes for motor speech deficits could be poor or missing dentition, decreased lingual range of motion, weak labial seal, or difficulty blowing up cheeks or kissing.

Sample Milestone Score with Interventions

Annie was a 4½-year-old preschooler whose oral repertoire included open-mouth vowels with spare consonants (e.g. MMA, baa) while playing. While there were gross delays related to her preference for play, she would be found producing the /ahh/ vowel most days as she jumped around the room grabbing items off the table and walking away. Since Annie's baseline speech sound production was mostly vowels, we worked on environmental noises and exclamations first with cause and effect toys (e.g. pound a ball), exclamations which I modeled for her were "oops!" "uh- ohhh!" along with basic nursery rhymes which we sang together while Annie bounced on her favored ball. I had found that when a child enjoying physical movement, often their speech sound production would increase while they are bouncing, swinging, jumping, etc.; so this was paramount to incorporate into our sessions together.

Area of Intervention: CVs (Environmental Noises)

Targeted intervention: This involves having the child bounce on a ball while practicing "ma" babbling, integrating movement to enhance the activity. During this exercise, the clinician engages in face-to-face interaction, encouraging the child to maintain eye contact to continue the bouncing. The gross motor movement from bouncing is intended to positively influence the fine motor movements involved in oral motor skills. Gross motor movements are movements of the larger extremities (e.g. legs, arms); whereas fine motor movements are the movements of the smaller body structures (e.g. lips, tongue, fingers).

Important Collaborative Measures

When there is a concern related to an oral motor apraxia, I will always reach out to the occupational therapist as well as physical therapist to see how the child's further fine and gross motor is impacted. Additional collaborations, particularly with an occupational therapist (OT), have proven beneficial, as these coworkers can assist with sensory deficits the child may have as well as desensitization of tolerance to more physical prompts for placement cues and articulation productions.

Preferred Methods and Procedures

While I do not have prompt training, the entire PROMPT program makes clinical sense regarding motor programming and coordination stimulation. I have always been an "all hands on deck" advocate regarding multisystem assistance for deficit areas. Therefore, when I have a child who has childhood apraxia of speech, I will refer to a PROMPT trained clinician to target their apraxia. The PROMPT institute, is an organization which provides a curriculum which trains clinicians on "hands-on tactile-kinesthetic input and emphasizes the need to integrate this into a holistic therapy approach" (The Prompt Institute, n.d.).

There are other programs out there, such as Kaufman cards with her associated training, which break down the interventions related to the complexity and positioning of vowels and consonants to each other. Nancy Kaufman is a speech-language pathologist who developed the Kaufman Speech to Language Protocol (K-SLP) as an evidence-based assessment and treatment approach for children with speech sound disorders, expressive language deficits and childhood apraxia of speech (Kaufman, 2024).

For those of my colleagues who need the means or resources to access the abovementioned training or further continuing education, I advise working with the level of complexity rule. A recommendation would be to target open mouth vowels over fricatives and speech sound blends, as the latter is later developing. Many consider this a more 'traditional' method to targeting speech sound and coarticulation productions, however; it supports the advancement from basic skills to skills which require increased complexity.

From more of a dysarthric speech perspective, many of the methods are geared toward compensatory strategies WHILE sequencing through advancing levels of complexity. A few compensatory strategies that I have utilized include slowing the rate of speech purposefully with over-articulation of speech sounds in words and phrases, allowing wait time for patients to formulate ideas as they put in effort to produce their sentences among others, and adequate breathing and respiratory support practices. Abovementioned middle schooler and I worked on 'practicing' classroom presentations prior to the actual event, to work on inserting 'pauses' to breath and support his 'voice.'

Motor Speech Progressions

Complexity of Coarticulation	*Acquired? Y/N, Emerging*
Vowels	
CV's (animal sounds/ environmental noises)	
CVC's (simple words)	
Multisyllabic words	
1+ word utterances	
Sentence length	

References

Kaufman, N. (2024, April 16). *Kaufman seminars & materials*. Kaufman Children's Center. https://www.kidspeech.com/meet-nancy-kaufman/

The Prompt Institute. (n.d.). The PROMPT institute. https://promptinstitute.com/

9   Speech Sounds and Phonological Norms

Speech sound errors, or articulation norms, are the areas where most parents and educators send students our way for referrals and requests. Refrain from downplaying the importance of articulatory accuracy and its potential impacts on phonological processes and implications. The speech sound development norms correlate with articulatory complexity. The bilabials (e.g. b, m, p) are expected to develop sooner than interdentals (e.g. voiced and voiceless 'th'). This particular knowledge and resource can especially help us in meetings when it comes to qualifying children for services and determining important short- and long-term goals related to a child's current level of articulatory functioning.

I also have included typical phonological process errors and their age of extinction for clinical reference. While articulation and phonological process' and disorders are extensively researched with particular emphasis on process' and procedures to assist with accurate speech sound attainment (e.g. prompt, dynamic systems, cyclical approach) – this portion is mainly included to provide a general understanding of where a child is performing in relation to motor speech complexity.

I would be remiss if I didn't acknowledge that different languages utilize different speech sounds. The speech sound norms listed in this chart are based on English language learners and not on other languages. I can provide an example of how it can be relevant and helpful to know general speech sound production across languages. I was referred to a child through the SST (student support team) to a child who speaks Gujarati at home as their first language. The parents were concerned about the child's 'd' and 'g' sound production. Before providing any insight into this area, I spoke with an old graduate school professor of mine who is fluent in this language – ensuring that the speech sound is utilized in the native language first and foremost. After inquiry, it determined that this speech sound should be mastered by the child's age (7) and utilized in both languages. While I was not able to attain a detailed speech sound acquisition chart for this child's native language, I was able to determine by complexity of the

DOI: 10.4324/9781003491842-9

language and it's other sounds and the discrepancy between the child now (7 years old) and the age in which a typical Gujarati speaker would learn this language – that this error was indeed abnormal, even in her native language.

Causes of Deficiencies

Common causes for such deficits could include certain syndromes (e.g. Down's), structural anomalies such as cleft lip or palate, differences in dentition (e.g. a child who utilizes a pacifier), and/or lack of explicit models of manner and production of speech sounds.

In the United States, we are very familiar with the Goldman Fristoe Test of Articulation (GFTA) (Goldman & Fristoe, 2015), which is utilized to stimulate all English speech sounds in different positions of words as well as sentences. So many children will receive standard scores in the 50's or below, leaving many perplexed on 'where to begin' intervention. This is where various methods can be utilized to determine which speech sounds to get the most 'bang for your buck.' While there is importance in articulation of speech sounds in a child's name (as the relevance and practicality is there). There are simply some speech sounds that are harder to co-articulate and thus, the accuracy can be impeded based on a child's current abilities. I have had a lot of children who have later acquisition sounds in their names (e.g. the 'r' consonant sound in Riley, Ryan), however, many of these children not only do not have the /r/ phoneme in their repertoire, but they do not even have a /k/ or /g/ or earlier acquisition sounds. This is where clinical judgment or complexity is weighed.

Sample Milestone Score with Interventions

Sam
4.5-year-old/male
Sam was a 4½-year-old boy who attended the local universal prekindergarten (UPK) in New York. Of course, his teachers noted his difficulty with the 'r' sound–a speech sound which we hear complaints about frequently from teachers and parents. However, after listening to Sam in the classroom, it was evident that he did not have the /f/ sound and would replace it with the /t/ – pronouncing /flower/ as /towa/, in fact his intelligibility was most impacted by the lack of 'v' and 'f' sounds than his 'r' errors. While Sam was of such a young age, tackling the 'r' phoneme did not make sense from an intelligibility or age/complexity standpoint. We targeted the 'f' and 'v' sounds first, as they were more visual and he had great eye contact and was responsive to cueing. Sam's parents soon reported that they

understood more than 85% of his speech. After explaining the visual and articulatory complexity of the /r/ sound to his parents and teachers, they agreed that it should be targeted later in his therapy.

Charles
8-year-old/male
Charles first came to me when he was in third grade having parents who were disgruntled over his speech sound errors which were pervasive. Charles was an articulate little boy (in that he had a LOT to say, and exhibited healthy receptive and expressive language skills). The way in which he wasn't articulate was with the production of his 'backed' sounds. Charles could not get the 'd' or 'g' phonemes into his repertoire. This led to him making comments during our speech group on "da titty tat" (instead of "the kitty cat") and he was of the age where his peers were poking fun at these pervasive errors. While Charles exhibited further difficulties with the voiced and voiceless 'th' and 'r's the phonological process of fronting his 'backed' sounds had the greatest impact on Charles. We began every treatment session with ALL the cues I could possibly employ to assist with the production of a backed sound, up to and including having him lay on the ground for accurate backed placement of the tongue. Eventually, Charles was able to produce these sounds in isolation and then with a segmentation approach. While it was "a long road" to correct phonological production and extinction of the phonological process of 'fronting,' Charles' speech was approximating a typical 8-year-old.

Important Collaborative Measures

Collaboration at the articulation level should include the student's teacher, particularly literacy. The reason why collaboration with a literacy expert is important is due to the potential phonological implications of articulation or phonological errors. As a side note, if a child's speech sound errors are impacting them phonetically (through reading or writing), this can generally qualify a student for intervention in the academic setting.

The first order when addressing speech sound errors is the child distinguishing between correct and incorrect production. The concern would be a child not hearing the difference between the sounds himself and this impacting his reading and writing. As you can see in this instance, there is a clear correlation between the two regarding speech sound production. As related to what a child is hearing, a consultation with an audiologist and full hearing screening is recommended. Remember the 'speech banana' we referred to in graduate school? If you are not aware of it, it is a visual representation of every speech sound in the English language as it relates to the frequency of sound it makes. I will reference below a link for your viewing. The speech banana illustrates where specific hearing loss can impact speech sounds! The most apparent difference would be that of the higher frequency sounds (e.g. /sh/ /th/). When a child cannot hear such sounds, their production will be voiced or distorted.

Preferred Methods and Procedures

Various articulation therapy methods are employed; I love to start with distinguishing between the sounds, oral feedback, and further utilization of mirrors for direct models of sounds with emphasis on articulatory production and distinct training of production.

When we are addressing phonological processes,' I target the process based on two differing areas – its impact on intelligibility of speech and the coarticulatory complexity of the speech sounds in that process. A clear example of this would be targeting the phonological processing of final consonant deletion for a 4-year-old before targeting the phonological process of gliding.

During treatment planning, I will utilize a multi-modal approach of increasing complexity to assist with correct speech sound production. In order: auditory discrimination (or minimal pairs), placement and manner training for correct production (with a mirror), sound in isolation, sound in differing positions at the word level, sounds in phrases, sentences, conversation. However, it is not a 'one size fits all' in our field, and sometimes, if a child's name starts with a speech sound in error, I will often target that speech sound, as it is client specific and relevant.

This particular section is for clinician reference to probe further with formalized articulation assessments.

Age of Mastery	Consonant Sounds	Acquired (y/n)
2:0–2:11	/b, n, m, p, h, w, d/	
3:0–3:11	/g, k, f, t, ng, j/	
4:0–4:11	/v, dge(judge), s, ch, l, sh, z/	
5:0–5:11	/r, voiceless th(think), ge (television)/	
6:0–6:11	/voiced th(with)/	

(Crowe, 2020)

Level of mastery
Zone of intervention
Age expectation

Phonological Process	Description	Age of Elimination (Years)	Exhibited (Y/N)
Velar assimilation	Nonvelars change to velars (due to their proximity to velars in the word), e.g. /guck – duck/	3	
Nasal assimilation	Non-nasal sounds change to nasals (due to their proximity to nasal sounds in the word), e.g. nunny – bunny	3	
Final consonant deletion	Deletion of the final consonant of a word, e.g. bu – bus	3	
Stopping	Fricative or affricate is replaced with a stopped sound, e.g. pun – fun	3–5 (depending on sounds)	
Fronting	Sounds made in back of mouth (velar) replaced with sounds produced in front of mouth, e.g. tar – car	4	
Deaffrication	Affricate replaced with fricative, e.g. ship – chip	4	
Cluster reduction	Consonant cluster is simplified with a single consonant, e.g. top – stop	4–5	
Weak syllable deletion	Unstressed/weak syllable in a word is deleted, e.g. nana – banana	4	
Gliding	Liquid sounds (/r/, /l/) replaced with glide (/w/ /j/), e.g. wabbit – rabbit	6–7	

(Bauman-Waegler, n.d.)

References

Bauman-Waengler, J.A. (2012). *Articulatory and phonological impairments.* New York: Pearson Higher Education.

Bernthal, J., Bankson, N.W., & Flipsen, P., Jr. (2013). *Articulation and phonological disorders.* New York: Pearson Higher Education.

Bauman-Waegler, J.A. (n.d.). *Selected phonological processes (patterns).* American Speechk-Language-Hearing Association. https://www.asha.org/practice-portal/clinical-topics/articulation-and-phonology/selected-phonological-processes/

Crowe, K., & McLeod, S. (2020, November). Children's English consonant acquisition in the United States: a review. *American Journal of Speech- Language Pathology, 29*(4), 2155–2169. https://doi.org/10.1044/2020_AJSLP-19-00168.

Goldman, R., & Fristoe, M. (2015). *Goldman-Fristoe test of articulation 3.* GFTA-3. https://www.pearsonassessments.com/store/usassessments/en/Store/Professional-Assessments/Developmental-Early-Childhood/Goldman-Fristoe-Test-of-Articulation-3/p/100001202.html

Peña-Brooks, A., & Hegde, M.N. (2015). *Assessment and treatment of speech sound disorders in children: A dual-level text.* Austin, TX: PRO-ED.

Shipley, K.G., & McAfee, J.G. (2016). *Assessment in speech-language pathology: A resource manual.* Boston, MA: Cengage Learning.

10 Swallowing and Feeding Milestones

Depending on when you attended graduate school for communication sciences and disorders has a significant impact on the scope and exposure you attained regarding pediatric feeding and swallowing. I can recall one pediatric dysphagia lesson in my graduate experience, of course, it was in the dysphagia course. However, my more intensive and hands-on pediatric feeding and swallowing experience came while I was 'on the job' working for early intervention in New York City. You have or will hear much overlap between speech-pathology and occupational therapy and our scopes of practice, regarding pediatric feeding and swallowing. I believe that, when we speak about true dysphagia and what is involved with modifications and interventions, a speech-language pathologist is covered in this' scope.' However, when we speak about more textural aversions, this is likely where more intense collaboration occurs between ourselves and our occupational therapy counterparts. Either way, the logical progression of a child's swallow and feeding is a topic many fellow speech-pathologists, OTs (occupational therapists), and parents approach me with. These milestones make sense about the maturity and complexity of the chew and swallow (as it can relate to oral motor control and the basis for speech production). What I find particularly interesting and important is how postural support (e.g. sitting independently) affects a baby's readiness to start solids. These milestones are essential for us to know about anatomy and positioning for safe feeding and swallowing, and they are also crucial for parents to know when introducing their children to new foods and textures.

Following my immersion in the 'feeding world' as it related to my work as an early interventionist, I have to admit I had found a textbook specifically designed for pediatric feeding to be immensely helpful. However, having a solid base of adult dysphagia clients, there were certain methods and considerations that were parallel. For one, aspiration can and does occur no matter what the age! For another, it often helps to start from the beginning and advance slowly particularly if an event has occurred rendering our clients unable to consume food by mouth as they

DOI: 10.4324/9781003491842-10

usually would. The main concept to think about here and have in the back of your mind as you glance over these is the parallel between fine motor and gross motor movements and a chew and swallow. Therefore, if a child (let's say) has a cranial nerve damage impacting her unilaterally (on one side), you can expect to see deficits not only orally but with their hands and other extremities.

Causes of Deficiencies

Deficits related to swallowing and feeding are typically brought up to speech-pathologists, as parents are concerned about what their child is and is not eating. However, a more obvious example would be a 4-year-old only eating yogurt and drinking bottles in a preschool program. This can span to a child who is rigid in his acceptance of different foods, only selecting food in dull color (e.g. crackers, bread, corn) or certain textures (e.g. cookies, chips).

Common causes for deficits can range anywhere, from anatomical anomalies to specific comorbid diagnoses, such as children on the autism spectrum (who often exhibit sensory deficits related to feeding).

At about 7 years into the field, I had a child who was diagnosed with Moebius syndrome. Having been assigned the case I quickly searched for information on the disease so I would "know what I was walking into" before our first session which was held during dinner time. For those of you unfamiliar with Moebius syndrome, it is a disorder in which the facial nerve is damaged during a child's birth. There appeared to be a great deal of ambiguity related to when and if the nerve would recover bilaterally, or if the damage was permanent. This case, in particular, is one which stood out to me, as we worked progressively to wean her from a very narrow 'Dr Browns' nipple spout, to a normal bottle and eventual cup drinking. The abovementioned case is one, in particular, where I think of as clear 'dysphagia' and not sensory-based intervention, thus the need for a feeding therapist (as opposed to being in an occupational therapists 'wheelhouse'). For those interested, I will reference Dr. Brown's products below; they offer varying nipples for different concerns related to feeding and swallowing.

Yet another child whom I was referred to in early intervention was only 5 months of age when I first walked into their apartment to treat him for 'feeding deficits.' I do feel that my history in working with adult dysphagic patients assisted me in this particular case as, while there was concern about his swallowing of foods, the child was primarily non-mobile and unable to hold himself up on the floor or hold his head up. While this case was complicated, as there were obvious comorbidities at play; I was adamant about pushing a formal modified barium swallow study (MBSS) and most of these sessions were related to the positioning of the child while he was being fed (e.g. NOT reclined) and determining the amount of liquid which he could tolerate at a time from the bottle.

Our work with pediatric feeding and swallowing is very important for the children and families that we serve. While there is a social aspect of sharing food and feeding others across cultures, there is an inherent need for parents to feel like they are helping their child thrive from a nutrition perspective. While the below-mentioned milestones do provide the typical age expectancies for such feeding and swallowing skills, know that they follow the sequence of complexity and, in some cases, can be utilized to progress our older clients toward a more 'solid' and unrestricted diet as well.

From a broader perspective, proper feeding and swallowing is a safety issue with both our pediatric and adult populations. Risk factors for dysphagia can include poor nutrition and hydration, aspiration, pneumonia, and even death. Therefore, we need to take our methods and procedures seriously and ensure our interventions are anatomically and physiologically based. When in doubt, complete your own research in areas of intervention, I will cite the textbook at the end of this chapter that I found particularly helpful when I began providing swallowing and feeding interventions with the early intervention population (children from birth through 3 years of age).

Sample Milestone Score with Interventions

Jared
4-year-old/male
Jared was a 4-year-old boy who is very mobile. He often preferred drinking his bottle while taking breaks from jumping around the classroom. He will take yogurt as spoon-fed by an adult. He will additionally, at times, attempt to escape from sitting at the table with peers while they were eating the state provided lunches. Jared would not even touch or look at the food on his plate and would pull his face away from a spoon presented to his mouth with a new or advanced texture.

Area of intervention – Cup drinking, eating mashed food, finger feeding.

Interventions – When advancing a child's food repertoire I ensure that I am explaining the basis to parents and educators. The idea that a child would go from primarily bottle drinking to eating solid foods overnight is quite the jump. Therefore, I briefly described to Jared's parents how we are going to 'warm up' their son to more advanced tastes and textures by exposing him to those newer stimuli slowly and succinctly. We started with utilization of a textured spoon to dip in puree, giving to the student to suck off and explore, and dipping the feeder into mashed bananas. During these sessions, we noted that Jared was able to lick and explore the feeder and even munch on mashed banana that was in the feeder. We also discovered he could drink from a straw, as he took a classmate's juicy juice and commenced sipping from it. This is where we introduced the Honey Bear straw cup, which assists with the inter oral pressure. While Jared was progressing through and toward solid foods, he was accepting the preferred milk via straw cup, a clear success and step in the right direction.

Sal
5-month-old/male
Sal was referred to my services under the early intervention division for "feeding difficulties." After conducting an attempted oral motor examination on Sal, much of his feeding skills were equivalent to a child between 2 and 4 months of age. Sal exhibited a flexed posture while feeding and remained partially stiff while his nanny presented the bottle to him. Sal was unable to sit up without assistance at all and did not always place his hand on the bottle during meals but instead pulled his head away. According to his presentation, Sal was performing well below age expectations but from a broader perspective, I was mainly concerned about the red flags that are associated with dysphagia and potential penetration or aspiration. Sal cried prior to feedings, would gurgle on the milk and further laryngeal elevation was not noticed during feeding. My first step in intervention included education of the caregivers on safe swallowing and feeding, up to and including the importance of reading a child's body language during mealtimes (Morris, 2000). Of course, a referral was put in with 'red flags' written to the attending physician for a formal modified barium swallow study. My interventions included proper positioning during mealtimes, altering the amount of liquid that was presented to the child and checking his swallow/suck pattern during the meal. While Sal's parent's 'goals' were to have their son 'eating solids,' this was a clear example of comparison to the typical development of swallow, a child was far below standards and expectations. It was my duty to assist in not only family and caregiver education but also methods to employ and collaborate with other healthcare professionals to provide this little one with the help he needed.

Important Collaborative Measures

As noted in one of my abovementioned case studies, collaboration with physicians is IMPERATIVE when we are addressing complex swallowing and feeding cases. When we are addressing dysphagia and concerns related to the safety of a client's swallow, there needs to be medical support and backing to coordinate next steps with families. I have referred patients to have diagnostic instrumentation conducted to visualize a swallow and further identify modifications and maneuvers that can be employed to assist in safe and pleasurable feeding and swallowing. Formal diagnostic instrumentation include/s modified barium swallow study (MBSS) and the Fiberoptic Evaluation of Swallowing (FEES) test. The modified barium swallow study is a specialized x-ray that allows the speech-language pathologist and radiologist to test your mouth, throat and esophagus while being presented with food and liquids. The flexible endoscopic evaluation of swallowing (FEES) passes an endoscope transnasally which permits the speech-language pathologist to identify abnormal swallow function and identify anatomical landmarks and abnormalities. Both formal evaluations permit the speech-language pathologist to identify areas of deficits in a client's swallow 'in real time' and make recommendations for interventions and change in diet (as necessary). It is to be noted that both of the above-mentioned tests can and are performed on children.

Since we require adequate swallow and breath collaboration, there are instances where a respiratory therapist is necessary to add to your team of collaborators when addressing a client's swallowing.

This area can significantly benefit from ongoing collaboration with the child's pediatrician and an occupational therapist and physical therapist. The collaboration between all three disciplines assists the child with gross motor (postural control) to assist with appropriate positioning during intake, fine motor (pincer grasp), and sensory aversions. There is often overlap between our disciplines, making collaboration an excellent way to troubleshoot and gain insight into other areas of a child's development to reach collective goals related to feeding and swallowing. My favorite approach to feeding aversions or rigidity is the food-chaining approach. Food chaining is a method which gradually enables a child to try new foods that are similar to the foods they currently enjoy. This approach requires a current feeding inventory and analyzes similarities which range from colors of foods to textures to tastes.

Preferred Methods and Procedures

Favorite intervention methods for feeding and swallowing treatment include the food chaining approach, successive approximation, and exposure therapy. While you note that I have mentioned the above methods, one can easily look at Arvedson's milestones, as listed below and utilize the methods to guide a child from where they are currently functioning to a more appropriate and complex oral intake.

The below milestones from Arvedson (2006), which reference the gross motor development that is needed to support those intricate fine motor movements of the articulators and swallowing mechanisms for the youngest of clients we see.

Note you will see a parallel between a child's gross motor development and maturity and their readiness for solids (Arvedson, 2006).

Age	Acquired skills	Acquired (Y/N)
2–6 months	Hand on bottle during feeding	
4–6 months	Maintains semi-flexed posture	
6 months	Sitting with support	
4–6 months	Semi-flexed posture during feeding	
6–9 months (transitory feeding)	Sitting independently for time	
6–9 months	Self-oral stimulation (mouthing hands and toys) Spoon feeding (thin, smooth puree) Suckle pattern (initially suck, swallow) Both hands hold bottle Pincer grasp (crawling on all fours) Finger feeding (introduced) Vertical munching (dissolvable solids) Prefers parents to feed	
9–12 months (first steps, cruising along furniture)	Cup drinking	
	Eats lumpy mashed food Finger feeding (dissolvable solids) Rotary chew action Assisting with spoon feeding	
12–18 months (refined gross and fine motor skills)	Self-feeding (grasps spoon with whole hand)	
	Holds cup with both hands Drinking with 4–5 consecutive swallows Holding and tipping bottle	
> 18–24 months	Swallowing with lip closure Self-feeding predominates Chewing varied range of food textures Up and down tongue movements More precise chew pattern	
24–36 months	Circulatory jaw rotations Chewing with lip closure Holds cup with one hand Open cup drinking w/o spillage Uses fingers to fill spoon Eats wide range of solids Independent feeding – using fork	

Level of mastery
Zone of intervention
Age expectation

References

Arvedson, Joan C. (2006). Developmental milestones and feeding skills birth to 36 months. https://www.nature.com/gimo/contents/pt1/fig_tab/gimo17_T3.html

Dr. Brown's Baby. (n.d.). *Dr. Brown's baby bottles.* https://www.drbrownsbaby.com/product-category/baby-bottles/

Lowsky, D. (2000). *Ark's bear bottle kit for straw drinking.* ARK Products, LLC. https://www.arktherapeutic.com/arks-bear-bottle-kit-for-straw-drinking/

Morris, S.E., Klein, M.D., & Satter, E. (2000). Pre-*feeding skills: A comprehensive resource for mealtime management.* Pro-ed.

11 Social-Emotional Milestones

The social stages are the most miraculous of many of the developmental stages of typical children. Scanning through these stages from infancy (e.g. smiles back at caregivers in infancy) makes us think how inherently important social connection is for humans. When describing social-communication and deficits, I speak about 'pragmatics' and, specifically, "the practice of speech and language." Our need to be seen and connect with our caregivers is inherent for most, whereas, for some, it needs to be fostered and developed through explicit intervention and guided cueing. You will notice that the social communication milestones also include carryover between Piaget's stages (e.g. development of object permanence). This is the area of development where speech therapists can utilize or foster a child's desire for human connection by interacting with our children based on where they are currently functioning. Such areas of distinction include cause and effect related to interactions (e.g. vocalizes to gain attention), emotional responses to others (e.g. fear of strangers), following rules, and embedding requests. When we are intervening with a much older child who does not have some of these baseline social stages (e.g. a sixth grader who does not attain eye contact for long enough to read facial cues), we are really speaking of its relevance to reading the emotional states of others, which is, arguably an important skill to have regarding communication.

Areas of Deficit

Deficits in social communication could include disinterest in others, behavior that is not interactional in nature (e.g. lining up cars instead of engaging in taking turns pushing to parent), and monotone in voice, to list a few. A common cause for such a deficit can indicate a child who is on the autism spectrum. The main characteristic of such a disorder includes decreased social interactions. To expand upon this, these social interactions

DOI: 10.4324/9781003491842-11

require the ability to 'read' other's emotions, body language, and a desire to interact with their environment.

Sample Milestone Score with Intervention

Jack and Jill were very premature twins when I was called into their Tribeca apartment in downtown Manhattan to provide early intervention speech therapy. They were cute as 'buttons' but both had speech which could be described as open mouth vowel vocalizations with appropriate inflection (e.g. with a loud noise that resembled 'hello' as I entered the apartment).

   Child's current stage: gains attention by vocalizing

   Zone of mastery: practicing vocal inflection

   Targeted intervention: Shaping vocalization to a functional word or exclamation (e.g. "hey!" or "look!"), engaging in vocal play while reading a book, or interacting by showing the child how to vary their inflection (e.g. the big bad wolf story with changing your vocal quality and tone) and directly modeling 'bye!' when their parent leaves the room or leaving – waiting (via expectant pause) for the child to repeat. I had additionally worked on exclamations and basic sounds to shape such vocalizations (e.g. ba-ba, moo- moo) with associated /Old McDonald/ manipulatives. This is where my childhood nursery rhyme file folders came in handy, rattling off familiar songs (e.g. five little ducks) and waiting for a more appropriate verbal approximation of the last word or sound in the series.

Important Collaborative Measures

Regarding referrals and collaboration, a referral and collaboration for applied behavioral analysis (ABA) therapy or specialized instruction can be profoundly beneficial when a child is not engaged in age-appropriate social stages. They will often discreetly target such skills as 'eye contact' and copying movements (e.g. hand over hand for 'give me' sign language). A psychologist is another professional to collaborate with regarding a child's social-emotional development as they can often determine the nature of the child's emotional state and identify if other comorbidities are existent.

Preferred Methods and Procedures

When we are speaking about social and emotional milestones which are expected at an early age, this is where 'getting on a child's level' is paramount. If a baby is immobile or with limited mobility. I will bring in a large mirror so we can imitate facial expressions in the mirror (e.g. sticking tongue out, blowing blueberries), as well as over accentuating oral movements and facial expressions. The mirror provides feedback for the child and increased personal engagement with the therapist (and parent) who can assist in making that emotional connection.

As you will notice, the below-mentioned social-emotional milestones incorporate facial expressions as well as body gestures and responses to others. Suggesting that attachment and interactions drive children at such a young age (of nearly 2 months to 12 months of age). Many of the below-mentioned milestones are, arguably, precursors to verbal expression (expressive language) milestones, as they are interactive in nature and can serve the same purpose of communicating nonverbally (CDC's Developmental Milestones, 2022).

Social interaction	Typical Age of acquisition	Mastered Y/N
Smile at people	2 months	
Can briefly calm selves (sucking on hands)	2 months	
Try to look at parents	2 months	
Smile spontaneously at people	4 months	
Enjoying playing with others (can cry when stops)	4 months	
Copy some movements and facial expressions (e.g. frowning)	4 months	
Know familiar faces (and strangers)	6 months	
Respond to others emotions	6 months	
Like to look at self in mirror	6 months	
Fear of strangers	9 months	
Cry when parents leave	1 year	
Verbalize for attention (repeat words or sounds)	1 year	
Play interactive games (e.g. 'pat a cake')	1 year	

Level of mastery

Zone of intervention

Age expectation

Reference

CDC's Developmental Milestones (2022, 17 August). *Centers for disease control and prevention.* Centers for Disease Control and Prevention. https://www.cdc.gov/ncbddd/actearly/milestones/index.html

12 Social Communication Benchmarks

The social communication milestones, as listed, can be considered healthy pragmatic skills. The quick and easy way I explain pragmatics to parents and fellow educators is the 'practice' of language as it relates to a child's social environment. While many language skills can easily be tested through formalized assessments, pragmatics are often more nuanced and can be at times hard to identify via formal methods. I cannot count the amount of conversations during Individualized Education Plan (aka IEP) meetings, with parents of school aged children in which a parent and teacher are seeing particular and specific pragmatic deficits in 'real time' that are not always demonstrated through formal evaluation meant to evoke pragmatic language concepts. As a result, I will often utilize a two-pronged approach for assessment and treatment of pragmatic deficits. If a standardized test is required (via the school district), I will administer this along with a questionnaire sent to parents and the child's educator to ascertain if the pragmatic skills are utilized across environments. This assists in not only leading to targeted intervention which can improve a child's pragmatic abilities both in and out of the classroom, but it also can stimulate a more collaborative approach in which the entire child's study team is working on pragmatic goals.

The benchmarks span through school ages of approximately 12 years, in which some of the higher-level pragmatic skills are targeted. These milestones are also helpful in listening comprehension, reading, and written language. A clear example would be using inferences in stories, which is expected between three and four years of age and can profoundly affect a third-grade child whose reading material requires inferencing skills. Social behaviors can additionally prove helpful for clinicians to know, as they can speak to general interests as they relate to development (e.g. showing fantasy schemes in play), as skilled therapy can cater to a child's interests. An example of catered intervention related to interest in fantasy would be utilizing Star Wars action figures, books, and activities with language expansion and recasting strategies. Language expansion refers to methods

DOI: 10.4324/9781003491842-12

utilized to take a child's language and expand its length and complexity, recasting strategies refer to taking an inaccurate language production and verbally repeating it with corrections.

The school-age-related milestones are not only insightful to learn and acknowledge when discussing higher-level language functioning and associated intervention but they can easily be carried over to the academic implications associated with a child not having such milestones. An example would be a child with inference deficits could have difficulty with reading (literacy skills) as often a third grade and older reading level requires a child to infer in order to demonstrate healthy reading comprehension. Such reference to inferential language, figurative language, and multiple meanings are all targets that speech-language pathologists work on when addressing pragmatic language skills with an older child.

Causes of Deficiencies

Deficits in higher-level pragmatics could look like a child who cannot maintain a topic and engages in a one-sided conversation, discussing only topics of personal interest without the knowledge or interest of their communicative partner. This described behavior must sound familiar, as a speech-language pathologist, as most of our children with Asperger's and/or autism spectrum behaviors exhibit difficulty in these metapragmatic skills.

When providing skilled intervention, as related to metapragmatics, there is value in explicit training (e.g. picture cards with associated visual double meanings) as well as trials with peers (e.g. turn-taking of conversational exchanges) during intervention sessions. In such sessions, speech therapists often look like more of a coach in which we are a go-between for our group sessions, providing faded visual and verbal cues to pass the conversational turn.

Sample Milestone Score with Interventions

Anna
Anna 10-year-old/female
Anna was a sweet, self-directed 10-year-old who had a love for everything related to 'Warrior Cats,' so much so that Anna had her neighborhood cat walking around their apartment while I was assessing her pragmatic language skills. Anna could maintain a topic with peers and adults (about cats) but had yet to extend the topic of conversation, nor did she understand when her peers used sarcasm. Anna's mom noted that due to her looming 'pms years' she was worried about Anna's lack of social prowess with peers.

Area of intervention: extending the topic of conversation, increasing the number of turns.

Example of intervention: We worked on visual and targeted turn-taking cues while practicing with peers and adults during intervention. With associated visual cues to assist with the flow of conversational exchange, encouraging Anna to look at the speaker while they were engaging with her so that she can 'read' their body language and respond so that they can make a connection over a joint interest. Intervention started in a setting of interest to Anna (e.g. that with an extraneous amount of Warrior Cat books and figurines) and later expanded to her local 'jump gym' that she enjoyed frequenting.

Ravi
5-year-old/male
Ravi was a quiet, happy 5-year-old who attended the universal pre-school. His social communication was much like those who present with an autism spectrum disorder. Ravi demonstrated scattered skills up to the 12–18 month expectancy. Meaning Ravi was able to demonstrate an increase in autonomy in the classroom, resistant control and showed anger or frustration (especially when you attempted to take away a toy car he was playing with).

Area of intervention: We addressed both the "use of single words to express intention" and "participates in verbal turn-taking."

Example of intervention: Speech-language sessions were set up, along with a visual schedule for Ravi to 'read' books with the clinician (primarily photo books), followed by completion of puzzles (with binary choice and 'show me' (insert item name). We worked on functional labels to request (e.g. 'car'?). After some time Ravi was able to demonstrate understanding of not only his visual schedule and our routine, but contingencies of first we 'work' and then we 'play' with desired object. Being forever short on space in our speech room, I share the room with another speech-language pathologist, whose child just so happened to like race cars as well. With the utilization of a 'race track' for the matchbox cars it took Ravi four sessions to functionally request a car from the peer and HAND him a car to demonstrate turn taking skills with a single word label. Of course, interventions and the amount of cues needed were faded over time (from maximum verbal/visual and tactile cues which looks like "give (name) the car" with associated hand-over-hand instruction; to minimal verbal/visual cues, "who's turn is it?").

Important Collaborative Measures

When we are addressing pragmatic deficits the key is collaborating ourselves across disciplines, therefore, collaboration with a child's teachers, sport instructors, occupational therapists, peers, siblings, and family all of whom are imperative to not only determine baseline but assist in a 'group' approach to target pragmatics.

To dial back the referrals, applied behavioral analysis (ABA) has proven to yield significant results when applied to children who have an autism diagnosis. Therefore, as soon as I have a clinical inclination that a child may be 'on the spectrum' I make a detailed referral to the pediatrician to approve ABA therapy IN the home.

When I mention the collaboration with various other disciplines such as teachers, coaches and family; this often entails speech coaching sessions, in which I demonstrate how many children with pragmatic deficits need to be explicitly taught certain social skills. I will send home information on the targets we have addressed in therapy that week so that parents are aware of ideas on how to carry those skills over at home. A very basic example of 'turn taking' as it can be carried over at home is the following: I had a child who loved to play soccer, he was QUITE good at the sport and loved to kick the ball around for hours in the backyard. At my request, his older brother and Dad worked on 'turn taking' with the ball as they practiced in the backyard. Not only did this skill assist in his gross motor skills and 'turn taking' but it prepared him for the higher level collaborative skills needed to play the actual game of soccer with teammates.

Preferred Methods and Procedures

If available, this is where a 'push-in' model can be so vital after explicitly teaching 'hypothetical' pragmatic skills. Often the common core as we call it in the United States (common core standards for grade levels) includes a collaborative component, which assists us in making pragmatic targets both academic and social in nature. I cannot count the number of times I have grabbed groups from an eighth grade class to work on a 'group project' where we can navigate the social skills 'in real and practical time.' Again, collaboration with teachers assists as most children feel comfortable with 'solo academic work' and can need a bit of a push to engage with others in the school setting.

There are times where the children I serve simply ask for a break from their classwork, at which time I utilize other teaching methods such as: board games, card games, video clips that require inference, as well as comic strips which require children to 'fill in the blank thought or speech bubble.' Board games are a wonderful way to incorporate not only turn-taking and social skills but following rules, utilizing problem solving skills and negotiation skills (executive functioning skills). My middle school students (students from sixth to eighth grade) particularly enjoyed playing Monopoly. Card games can vary from the most simple (e.g. Go Fish) to more complex (e.g. Apples to Apples). I have utilized the 'Apples to Apples' game countless times with my middle schoolers. Basically it is a game in which they have to pair their group of nouns with an adjective that is thrown for the players to 'play' the best 'match' that gains them points. I have utilized this game to not only target 'persuasive thoughts' but also writing and answering questions related to 'why.' There are various clips online that are targeted to address 'inferencing' but what I especially like about 'video learning' is that the children have to READ the facial expressions and body language of characters to ascertain the real meaning behind their actions. One of the last therapy activities I like to use with my children from kindergarten and up is the utilization of 'blank comic strips.' This permits them to use their creativity, within reason, to demonstrate understanding of pragmatics as they relate to reading visual cues.

Social Communication Benchmarks

Birth–12 months

Action	Acquired (Y/N)
Prefers looking at human face and eyes	
Prefers human voices	
Looks for source of sound	
Differentiates b/n tones of voice (angry/ friendly)	
Smiles back at caregiver	
Follows caregivers gaze	
Participates in preverbal vocal turn-taking	
Vocalizes to gain attention	
Demonstrates joint attention skills (sharing attention	
Uses gestures to make requests and direct attention	
Plays simple interactive games (peekaboo)	
Seeks comfort from caregiver	
Expresses feelings	
Develops object permanence	
Discriminates facial expressions	
Fear of strangers	
Relational memory develops (faces/ voies)	
Changes behavior to achieve goal	
Imitates gestures/oral movements	

12–18 months

Range of communicative intentions
  (requests, comments)
Brings objects to show caregivers
Requests via pointing and vocalizing
Gains attention by vocalizing
Practices vocal inflection
Says "bye" and other ritualized
  greetings
Protests by shaking head and
  saying "no"
Uses gestures with verbal language
Demonstrates awareness of the social
  value of speech
Responds to others' speech by giving
  eye contact
Demonstrates sympathy, empathy and
  sharing nonverbally
Shows joy, fear and anger
Increase in autonomy
Resists control
Co-regulates interactions

(Wellman, 2011)

18–24 months

Uses single words to express intention
Single and paired words to command,
  indicate possession and gain
  attention
Uses I, me, you, my and mine
Participates in verbal turn taking
  (limited turns)
Demonstrates simple topic control
Interrupts at syntactic junctures or in
  response to prosodic cues
Demonstrates secure and insecure
  attachment pattern
Exhibits emotion and behavioral
  regulation
Demonstrates increase in autonomy
Develops emerging implicit perceptual
  access reasoning
Shows daily routine schemes in play

24–36 months

Engages in short dialogues
Verbally introduces and changes topic
Expresses emotion
Begins to use language in
    imaginative way
Relates own experiences
Begins to include descriptive details to
    enhance listeners understanding
Uses attention-getting words
Clarifies and asks for clarification
Uses politeness terms or markers
Begins to demonstrate adaptation of
    speech to different audience/listeners
Can deceive and detect deception
Understands that others may feel
    differently than themselves
Follows rules
Shows common but not daily schemes
    in play (e.g. doctor, shopping)
Uses embedded requests

3–4 years (Adams, 2002)

Engages in longer dialogues
Anticipates next turn at talking
Terminates conversation; appropriately
    role-plays
Uses filers (e.g. "yeah" "okay") to
    acknowledge partners message
Begins code-switching and using
    simpler language when talking to
    very young children
Uses elliptical responses (e.g. "mommy
    went home, I didn't")
Requests permission
Begins using language for fantasies,
    jokes and teasing
Makes conversational repairs when not
    understood and correct others
Infers information from a story and
    infers indirect meanings
Uses primitive narratives – events
    follow from central core
Uses inferences in stories

4–5 years

Uses indirect requests; correctly uses
 deictic terms (e.g. this, that, there,
 here)
Uses twice as many effective utterances
 as 3-year-olds to discuss emotions and
 feelings
Uses narrative development characterized
 by unfocused chains – stories have
 a sequence of events but no central
 character or theme
Develops basic understanding of theory
 of mind, including judgment that
 another person may have a believe
 that differs from the truth
Shifts topics rapidly
Shows fantasy schemes in play
Understands that beliefs can result in
 predictable emotions
Understands that someone may feel the
 same way when experiencing a similar
 event
Uses comissives/promises

(Wellman, H.M., 2011)

School-age years (6–12 years)

Demonstrates increased understanding
 of theory of mind (predicting what
 one person is thinking about what
 another person is thinking or feeling;
 understands strategies to hide deceit,
 recognizes sarcasm)
Provides assistance and demonstrates
 altruism
Uses narrative development
 characterized by causally sequenced
 events using "story grammar"
Demonstrates improved conversational
 skills (e.g. topic maintenance, repair,
 increased number of turns)
Extends topic of conversation
Demonstrates refined social conventions
Demonstrates metapragmatic
 skills – child is able to think about
 social and conversational rules

(Continued)

(Continued)

Uses language for varied functions, including persuading and advancing one's opinion
Understands that people can feel multiple emotions at the same time
Practices increased self-regulation
Uses indirect requests
Uses inferential language
Uses ambiguous language (figurative)
Uses sarcasm
Uses double meanings (puns)

(Gard, 1993)

Level of mastery
Zone of intervention
Age expectation

References

Adams, C. (2002). Practitioner review: The assessment of pragmatics. *The Journal of Child Psychology and Psychiatry, 43*(8), 973–987. https://doi.org/10.1111/1469-7610.00226

Gard, A. et al. (1993). *Speech and language development chart* (2nd ed.). Pro-Ed.

Hwa-Froelich, D.A. (in press). *Social communication development and disorders* (2nd ed.). Taylor & Francis.

Russel, R.L. (2007). Social communication impairments: Pragmatics. *Pediatric Clinics of North America, 54*(3), 483–506. https://doi.org/10.1016/j.pcl.2007.02.016

Wellman, H.M., et al. (2011). Sequential progressions in a theory-of-mind scale: Longitudinal perspectives. *Child Development, 82*(3), 780–792. https://doi.org/10.1111/j.1467-8624.2011.01583.x

13 Brown's Stages of Morphological and Syntactic Development

Roger Brown (1973) was a researcher and author who provided a staged framework to understand normal expressive language development in English regarding a child's morphology and syntax. Generally, when we dive into Brown's stages, we perform a structural analysis of a child's language sample. The two areas analyzed in Brown's stages include morphology and syntax. Morphology is the area of grammar related to the structure or forms of words with one morpheme as a unit of meaning. In comparison, syntax is the rules governing combining words that form sentences. In particular, I reference Brown's stages related to expected MLU (or mean length of utterance) as an easy barometer when listening to a child speak for the first time. I generally tell parents that a child's MLU should correlate with their age, therefore giving a child who is 1.5 years old between 1–2 words per utterance. Brown's stages dive into the complexity and specific grammatical knowledge a child should acquire regarding language growth. This particular portion of the protocol can delineate a child's complexity of language models as related to their current functioning. They provide targets as the intervention progresses' based on their language stage and morphological structure.

When addressing speech and language deficits for older children, Brown's stages provide invaluable information related to their complexity of speech. Having spent a vast majority of my time as a working speech-language pathologist in the school setting, I can account for the goals as they relate to language complexity in the classroom. Brown's stages of morphological and syntactic development can be noted during actual speech but also during written language analysis. We often explicitly teach the grammatical rules to our written language learners in elementary school and up. What I like about Brown's stages is he speaks on MLU (or mean length of utterance) as it associates with each stage. I would like to expand upon the MLU briefly here, I will often tell parents that the general 'rule of thumb' for MLU is that it should correlate with a child's age, advancing

DOI: 10.4324/9781003491842-13

and growing as the child grows. Therefore, when a child hits 1 year old, they should be speaking in one-word utterances, and so forth. This can assist with quick intervention with a child, as a child who is 1 year old should be provided language models which are very label and vocabulary rich (e.g. 'dog' 'cookie' 'ball'); as opposed to what a lot of parents want to do, which is full out 'narration' (e.g. "look at that big, doggie, woof-woof, fluffy, he is running.") Do you see where a child who is at a 1.0 MLU could get 'lost in the woods' with such an elaborate language model? This is where our language scaffolding measures come into play, particularly with relation to a child's MLU.

The most apparent deficits in Brown's stages include a child with one-word utterances with no possessives of plurals, indicating the simplest morphological models. However, as a child progresses past the 1+ word labels, Brown's stages can demonstrate advancing linguistic complexity— these progress past pure labels to attributes, requests for more, and so on. When a child is non-verbal and utilizing augmentative and alternative communication (AAC) devices to communicate, the sentence and syntax structure can still be stimulated in the same developmental fashion to increase linguistic complexity.

Generally, a cause for deficits in lack of morphological complexity can be related to receptive language deficits. Suppose a child does not have the building blocks and understanding of language and the world around them. In that case, their language will be more simplistic and parallel their general understanding.

Sample Milestone Score with Interventions

Nala
4.5-year-old/female
Nala was a 4.5-year-old who attended our UPK classroom (universal pre-school) in the Upper West Side of Manhattan. She was always giggling and with a smile on her face. However, most of her language felt abbreviated, meaning her MLU was approximately 2.0 when I first met her, and she was just nearing 4 years of age. According to Brown's stages, Nala used appropriate agent+action (e.g. "Doggie go"), action+ object (e.g. "eat cookie"), but did not utilize prepositional phrases or present progressive endings (e.g. running).

Stage of Intervention: Stage II

Nala loved books, particularly books about fancy Nancy, since she herself liked wearing tutus over her brightly decorated leggings to 'match' her sparkly Keds. This is where utilization of literacy had proved paramount into intervention with Nala. We spoke about the actions Fancy Nancy was doing on the pages (embedded twirling, dancing, running, jumping) and further practiced these actions 'while' reading the book (in the speech room). We also addressed prepositional phrases by playing a 'hide and seek' game with my miniature Fancy Nancy dolly, taking turns giving 'clues' as to where she was hiding, or where she left her fancy crown. As you can see, the utilization of her current interests (anything FANCY) along with her current stage, and stage of intervention; made therapy and intervention planning a fun breeze.

Intervention: Book reading, pretend play, emphasis on asking 'what doing' questions with direct models, repetition, and practice.

Boys Group.

Group of three males between ages of 13–14 years of age.

For my speech-pathologists who are familiar with the group mandate setting you will appreciate this case in which I will term BG (for 'boys' group). Every one of the boys in this speech room was working on appropriate morphological and syntactic expressions both verbally and in their written language. The way I 'posed' our sessions to them was that we were "practicing grammatical rules that even Miss L needs to follow when writing an email to the principal." The boys in this group were performing in Brown's IV stage; they were able to utilize articles and regular past tense most of the time, where they fell apart 'so to say' was in Brown's V stage of morphological and syntactic development. It just so happened that my BG enjoyed playing games in speech, therefore, every few sessions I would get out the 'Apples to Apples' game which I had referenced in the previous chapter. With explicit targets related to certain areas of 'grammar for the day' they would 'share' their combinations utilizing grammatically correct phrases or sentences. We were able to practice 'grammar rules' in a fun and supportive environment, with visual aides to assist (e.g. sentence starters that were grammatically appropriate). Soon, my BG would self-correct while sharing a story of what was going on in the lunchroom that day utilizing appropriate morphological and syntactical word forms!

Important Collaborative Measures

Collaboration with a student's teacher is paramount when addressing advancing language complexity. In its most obvious forms, a child in preschool and kindergarten will begin to "write their own stories" and need to demonstrate understanding of text read aloud. This is where close collaboration with a child's teacher comes into effect. As it is essential to make language learning as hands-on as possible, a clear pre-literacy and dialogic approach to reading is also paramount to develop with intervention.

You will note that in the next section I will briefly touch on the importance of reading and literacy skills as a more 'passive' method to teach children linguistic complexity. I utilize this same method when I am making recommendations to parents during Individualized Education Plan (IEP) meetings. The easiest way to expose your child to new and advanced vocabulary is to get them interested in reading. This stands true for linguistic complexity, as children when children read they are provided a model of appropriate linguistic structure.

Preferred Methods & Procedures

Intervention to be utilized includes a child-led model, with language recasting, modeling, and expansion for intervention with younger children. Further dialogic reading approaches can be especially helpful when we are providing intervention to children who are of school age (kindergarten and up).

Dialogic reading is a method of reading and instilling pre-literacy skills in children by making the book more 'interactive.' It can be described as having an open conversation ABOUT the book with children (Zavala Iturbe, 2019). I have utilized this method and scaffolded it appropriately based on the level of the children which I am intervening with. For example, during my push-in sessions with the universal preschoolers, I will utilize prompts based on the pictures that accompany the text on the page, oftentimes leaving out the 'words on the page' entirely, to ensure that the child is engaged with the 'idea' of the story rather than the words. With my older children, I will utilize the methods in its entirety, touching on the dialogic C.R.O.W.D. prompts to expand the contents of the book. C stands for completion prompts, R for recall prompts, O for open-ended prompts, W for wh question prompts, and D for distancing prompts. I implore you to dive into the article cited here which covers the method of dialogic reading. This method can not only target higher-level linguistic skills (such as Brown's syntax and morphological structures below) but additionally vocabulary acquisition.

Brown's Stages

Stage	Age Range	MLU	Morphological Structure	Examples	Acquired?
I	15–30	1.75 (1.5–2.0 range)	Stage I Sentence Types	Nomination (that doggie) Negation (no juice) Recurrence (more cookie) Possession (my cookie) Attribution (big ball) Locative (cup table) Agent+ action (mommy go) Action+ object (hit ball) Agent+object (daddy truck)	
II	26–36	2.25 (2.0–2.5)	1. Present progressive (-ing ending on verbs) 2. In 3. On 4. -s plurals (regular plurals)	1. It going, falling off 2. In box, pussy in 3. On tree, birdie on head 4. My cars, two ties	
III	36–42	2.75 (2.5–3.0)	1. Irregular past tense 2. -s possessives 3. Uncontactable copula (the full form of the verb 'to be' when it's the only verb in a sentence)	1. Me fell down 2. Doggie's bone, mommy's hat 3. Are they there? Is it Allison?	
IV	40–46	3.5 (3.0–3.7)	1. Articles 2. Regular past tense (-ed endings on verbs) 3. Third person regular present tense	1. A book, the book 2. She jumped, he laughed 3. He swims, man brings	
V	42–52+	4.0 (3.7–4.5)	1. Third person irregular 2. Uncontractible auxiliary (the full form of verb 'to be' when it's an auxiliary verb in a sentence) 3. Contractible copula (shortened form of verb 'to be' when it's the only verb in sentence) 4. Contractible auxiliary (shortened form of verb 'to be' when it's an auxiliary verb in sentence)	1. She has, he does 2. Are they swimming? 3. She's ready. They're here 4. They're coming. He's going.	

(Miller, 2010)

Level of mastery
Zone of intervention
Age expectation

References

Brown, R. (1973). *A first language: The early stages.* London: George Allen & Unwin.

Miller. (2010, October). SLI guidelines. http://ioniaisd.pbworks.com/w/file/fetch/38468819/33MLU%20Chart.pdf (Accessed 11 December 2022).

Zavala Iturbe, C. (2019, April 18). *What is dialogic reading? | Cambridge English.* Cambridge English. https://www.cambridge.org/elt/blog/2019/04/18dialogic-reading/

Glossary of Terms

AAC Augmentative and alternative communication (AAC) device. An AAC device is typically in the form of a tablet or laptop that assists a client with speech or language impairments in communicating. There are varying 'types' of AAC including no-tech (gestures, writing, pointing), low-tech (pointing, drawing), and high-tech (iPad, tablet) (American Speech-Language-Hearing Association, n.d.).

ABA Stands for applied behavioral analysis, a method of treatment which is based on behavioral principles.

Anomia A word-finding deficit (inability to retrieve a word).

ASHA aka American Speech and Hearing Association – the professional association for speech – language pathologists; audiologists; and speech, language, and hearing scientists in the United States and internationally.

Aspiration When food or liquid enters an airway and eventually lungs.

Audiogram A chart which records the results from a series of hearing tests. The associated 'speech banana' is the speech sounds as they relate to Hz (hearing).

Binary choice Choice between two items.

Child-directed approach aka Child-led therapy, following the child's interests and allowing them to 'lead the way' during sessions.

Clinical Fellowship Year aka CF year; the first year a speech-language pathologist works in the field of speech-pathology in the United States in which they are supervised.

Common Core Standards The Common Core Standards Initiative (aka Common Core) is a multi-state educational initiative with the goal of increasing consistency across state education standards (Common Core State Standards Initiative, 2021).

Comorbidities When a person has more than one condition or disease at a time. Conditions described as such are often chronic or long-term conditions.

CVA   Cerebral vascular accident is the medical term for a stroke. This is when the blood flow to the brain is stopped either by a blockage or by rupture of a blood vessel (Ellis, 2018).

Dentition   Medical term for teeth.

Diadochokinetic rate (DDK)   A unit of measure utilized to assess, diagnose, and treat problems. Measures how quickly you can accurately repeat a series of rapid, alternating sounds (aka tokens). It is designed to test how well you make sounds in different parts of your mouth, tongue, and soft palate. These 'tokens' contain one, two, and three syllables e.g. 'puh,' 'puh-tuh,' 'puh-tuh-kah.' The DDK rate measures the repetition of sounds within a specific amount of time (Rice, 2017).

Dialogic reading   A method of reading which involves "having a conversation about a book" (Zavala Iturbe, 2019).

Executive functioning   Executive functioning are "mental processes that enable us to plan, focus attention, remember and juggle multiple tasks." Some of the areas that are encompassed in executive functioning include working memory, mental flexibility, and self-control (Center on the Developing Child at Harvard University, 2020).

Exposure therapy   A treatment developed to help people overcome things, activities, or situations that cause anxiety or fear (Yetman, 2021).

FEES   Passes an endoscope transnasally which permits the SLP to identify abnormal swallow function and identify anatomical landmarks and abnormalities.

Food chaining approach   Method that begins with feeding a child food that they like and making small changes to work toward expanding their repertoire to accept newer foods (Fishbein et al., 2006).

IEP   aka Individualized Education Program – a legal document under United States law that is developed for each child attending public school in the United States who needs special education services.

Intelligibility   The degree to which speech sounds can be understood by listeners (American Psychological Association, n.d.).

Intonation and inflection   When a person's voice rises and falls as they speak.

Joint attention   When one person purposefully coordinates their focus of attention with that of another person. "It involves two people paying attention to the same thing, intentionally and for social reasons" (UNC School of Medicine, n.d.).

Labial   Medical term for lips.

Labial seal   Refers to the lips closing in their entirety.

Lingual   Medical term for tongue.

Mand model   When a child expresses interest, you mand (e.g. verbally instruct or point) for the child to respond (Vanderbilt University, 2013).

MBS   The modified barium swallow study is a specialized x-ray that allows the speech-language pathologist and radiologist to test your mouth, throat, and esophagus while being presented with food and liquids.

Moebius syndrome   A "rare congenital (present at birth) condition that results from underdevelopment of the facial nerves that control some of the eye movement and facial expressions." It can impact the nerves responsible for speech, swallowing, and chewing (Johns Hopkins Medicine (2023).

Neuronal connections   The connection between neurons, one cell 'talking to another.'

Oral Motor Examination   A comprehensive examination conducted to evaluate the functioning of oral structures involved in swallowing and speech production; includes assessment of the lips, tongue, palate, jaw, and other relevant areas to identify any abnormalities or impairments (Baslpcourse.com, 2023).

Parkinson's disease   Parkinson's is a brain disorder that causes unintended or uncontrollable movements, such as shaking, stiffness, and difficulty with balance and coordination, and targets the nerve cells in the basal ganglia portion of the brain (National Institute of Aging, 2022).

PECS   Picture Exchange Communication System, augmentative/alternative communication system based on B.F. Skinner's book /Verbal Behavior/ and applied to behavior analysis. Utilization of specific prompting and reinforcement strategies leads to independent communication (Pyramid Educational Consultants, 2023).

Rett's syndrome   A "rare genetic neurological disorder which leads to severe impairments in speaking, eating, walking and breathing" (International Rett Syndrome Foundation, 2024).

SOS   Sequential Oral Sensory (SOS) feeding approach is a multidisciplinary approach to feeding, it encourages children to learn and explore food in a playful way that increases their comfort level with new textures gradually (SOS Approach to Feeding, 2024).

Successive approximation   aka shaping, "successive reinforcement of close and closer approximations to the target behavior" (Skinner, 1953).

UPK   Universal prekindergarten, which is provided to families in New York State.

References

About the Standards | Common Core State Standards Initiative. (2021). *About the standards.* https://www.thecorestandards.org/about-the-standards/

American Psychological Association. (n.d.). *APA dictionary of psychology.* https://dictionary.apa.org/speech-intelligibility

American Speech-Language-Hearing Association. (n.d.). *Augmentative and alternative communication (AAC).* American Speech-Language-Hearing Association. https://www.asha.org/public/speech/disorders/aac/

Baslpcourse.com. (2023, December 16). *How to do an oral mechanism exam.* BASLP COURSE. https://baslpcourse.com/how-to-do-an-oral-mechanism-exam/

Center on the Developing Child at Harvard University. (2020, March 24). *Executive function & self-regulation.* https://developingchild.harvard.edu/science/key-concepts/executive-function/

Cochlear. (2024, February 1). *What is an audiogram and how to read it.* https://www.cochlear.com/us/en/home/diagnosis-and-treatment/diagnosing-hearing-loss/understanding-the-audiogram.

Ellis, M.E. (2018, September 29). *Cerebrovascular accident: Symptoms, treatment, and prevention.* Healthline. https://www.healthline.com/health/cerebrovascular-accident#diagnosis

Fishbein, M., Cox, S., Swenny, C., Mogren, C., Walbert, L., & Fraker, C. (2006, April). Food chaining: a systematic approach for the treatment of children with feeding aversion. *Nutrition in Clinical Practice, 21*(2), 182–184. https://doi.org/10.1177/0115426506021002182. PMID: 16556929.

Individuals with Disabilities Education Act. (2017, July 12). *Sec. 300.320 definition of individualized education program.* https://sites.ed.gov/idea/regs/b/d/300.320

International Rett Syndrome Foundation. (2024, March 5). *What is rett syndrome?* https://www.rettsyndrome.org/about-rett-syndrome/what-is-rett-syndrome/

Johns Hopkins Medicine. (2023, March 8). *Moebius syndrome.* https://www.hopkinsmedicine.org/health/conditions-and-diseases/moebius-syndrome#:~:text=Moebius%20syndrome%20is%20a%20rare,for%20speech%2C%20chewing%20and%20swallowing.

National Institute of Aging. (2022). *Parkinson's disease: Causes, symptoms, and treatments | National Institute on Aging.* https://www.nia.nih.gov/health/parkinsons-disease/parkinsons-disease-causes-symptoms-and-treatments

Pyramid Educational Consultants. (2023, April 17). *PECS®: An evidence-based practice.* https://pecsusa.com/pecs/

Rice, S.C. (2017, March 31). *Diadochokinetic rate: Definition and patient education.* Healthline. https://www.healthline.com/health/diadochokinetic-rate

Skinner, B.F. (1953). *Method of successive approximation.* American Psychological Association. https://dictionary.apa.org/method-of-successive-approximations

SOS Approach to Feeding. (2024, February 23). *Feeding disorders in children.* https://sosapproachtofeeding.com/

UNC School of Medicine. (n.d.). *About joint attention.* https://www.med.unc.edu/healthsciences/asap/materials-1/about-joint-attention/

Vanderbilt University. (2013). *Intentional instruction: Instructional strategies.* The Center on the Social and Emotional Foundations for Early Learning. https://www.pyramidmodel.org/wp-content/uploads/2021/04/H2.8.pdf

Yetman, D. (2021, June 21). *Exposure therapy: Types, how it's done, and more.* Healthline. https://www.healthline.com/health/exposure-therapy

Yetman, D. (2022, April 4). *Comorbidity: Definition, types, risk factors, treatment & more.* Healthline. https://www.healthline.com/health/comorbidity

Zavala Iturbe, C. (2019, April 18). *What is dialogic reading? | Cambridge English.* Cambridge English. https://www.cambridge.org/elt/blog/2019/04/18/dialogic-reading/

References

The Administration for Children and Families. (2023). *Head start services*. https://www.acf.hhs.gov/ohs/about/head-start

American Psychological Association. (n.d.). *APA dictionary of psychology*. https://dictionary.apa.org/speech-intelligibility

American Speech-Language-Hearing Association. (n.d.). *Augmentative and alternative communication (AAC)*. https://www.asha.org/public/speech/disorders/aac/

Baslpcourse.com. (2023, December 16). *How to do an oral mechanism exam*. BASLP Course. https://baslpcourse.com/how-to-do-an-oral-mechanism-exam/

Bondy, A. (2023, April 17). *PECS®: An evidence-based practice*. Pyramid Educational Consultants. https://pecsusa.com/pecs/

Brown, R. (1973). *A first Language: The early stages*. London: George Allen & Unwin.

Dr. Brown's Baby. (n.d.). *Dr. Brown's baby bottles*. https://www.drbrownsbaby.com/product-category/baby-bottles/

Cochlear. (2024, February 1). *What is an audiogram and how to read it*. https://www.cochlear.com/us/en/home/diagnosis-and-treatment/diagnosing-hearing-loss/understanding-the-audiogram

Drew, C., & Cornell, D. (2023, October 11). *Parten's 6 stages of play in childhood, explained!* Helpful Professor. https://helpfulprofessor.com/stages-of-play/

Ellis, M.E. (2018, September 29). *Cerebrovascular accident: Symptoms, treatment, and prevention*. Healthline. https://www.healthline.com/health/cerebrovascular-accident#diagnosis

Goldman, R., & Fristoe, M. (2015). *Goldman-Fristoe Test of Articulation 3 (GFTA-3)*. https://www.pearsonassessments.com/store/usassessments/en/Store/Professional-Assessments/Developmental-Early-Childhood/Goldman-Fristoe-Test-of-Articulation-3/p/100001202.html

Greenspan, S. (2010). *What is floortime?* Home of DIR Floortime® (Floortime). https://www.icdl.com/floortime

The Hanen Centre | Speech and Language Development for Children. (2016). *The Hanen Centre: Speech and language development for children*. https://www.hanen.org/Home.aspx

International Rett Syndrome Foundation. (2024, March 5). *What is Rett Syndrome?* https://www.rettsyndrome.org/about-rett-syndrome/what-is-rett-syndrome/

Johns Hopkins Medicine. (2023, March 8). *Moebius syndrome.* https://www. hopkinsmedicine.org/health/conditions-and-diseases/moebius-syndrome# :~:text=Moebius%20syndrome%20is%20a%20rare,for%20speech%2C%20 chewing%20and%20swallowing.

Kaufman, N. (2024, April 16). *Kaufman seminars & materials.* Kaufman Children's Center. https://www.kidspeech.com/meet-nancy-kaufman/

Lowsky, D. (2000). *Ark's bear bottle kit for straw drinking.* ARK Products, LLC. https://www.arktherapeutic.com/arks-bear-bottle-kit-for-straw-drinking/

Mcleod, S. (2024a, February 1). *Albert Bandura's social learning theory in psychology.* Simply Psychology. https://www.simplypsychology.org/bandura.html

Mcleod, S. (2024b, February 1). *Vygotsky's zone of proximal development & scaffolding theory in psychology.* Simply Psychology. https://www.simplypsychology. org/zone-of-proximal-development.html

Miller. (2010, October). SLI Guidelines. http://ioniaisd.pbworks.com/w/file/ fetch/38468819/33MLU%20Chart.pdf. Accessed 11 December 2022.

Morris, S.E., et al. (2000). *Pre-feeding skills: A comprehensive resource for mealtime Development.* Austin, Texas, Pro-Ed.

National Institute of Aging. (2022). *Parkinson's disease: Causes, symptoms, and treatments | National Institute on Aging.* https://www.nia.nih.gov/health/ parkinsons-disease/parkinsons-disease-causes-symptoms-and-treatments

New York State Department of Health. (1993). *Department of Health: Early intervention program.* https://www.health.ny.gov/community/infants_children/ early_intervention/

Newsela. (n.d.). *Engage, support, and grow every learner.* https://newsela.com/about/ products/?utm_source=google&utm_medium=paid-search&utm_campaign= google-search-brand&utm_term=brand&gad_source=1&gclid=Cj0KCQjw_ qexBhCoARIsAFgBleueMqgNSW9sbhH4-HyZgF3S-9sEk39brv10ER4Sj- mAhXevuOgkFtNMaAiNYEALw_wcB

The PROMPT Institute. (n.d.). https://promptinstitute.com/

Rice, S.C. (2017, March 31). *Diadochokinetic rate: Definition and patient education.* Healthline. https://www.healthline.com/health/diadochokinetic-rate

Ruhl, C. (2023, August 28). *What is theory of mind in psychology?* Simply Psychology. https://www.simplypsychology.org/theory-of-mind.html

Skinner, B. F. (1953). *Method of successive approximation.* American Psychological Association. https://dictionary.apa.org/method-of-successive-approximations

SOS Approach to Feeding. (2024, February 23). *Feeding disorders in children.* https://sosapproachtofeeding.com/

Sussex Publishers. (2020). *Executive function.* Psychology Today. https://www. psychologytoday.com/us/basics/executive-function

UNC School of Medicine. (n.d.). *About joint attention.* https://www.med.unc.edu/ healthsciences/asap/materials-1/about-joint-attention/

Vanderbilt University. (2013). *Intentional instruction: Instructional strategies.* The Center on the social and emotional foundations for early learning. https://www. pyramidmodel.org/wp-content/uploads/2021/04/H2.8.pdf

Yetman, D. (2021, June 21). *Exposure therapy: Types, how it's done, and more.* Healthline. https://www.healthline.com/health/exposure-therapy

Yetman, D. (2022, April 4). *Comorbidity: Definition, types, risk factors, treatment & more.* Healthline. https://www.healthline.com/health/comorbidity

Appendix A
The Protocol by Stephanie LoPresti

I Introduction

    A Answering the 'why' behind the development of the protocol

    B Personal history behind the interest in merger between psychology and speech-language pathology service delivery and assessments

    C Brief overview of the zone of proximal development and discrepancy between where a child is currently performing and how they should be performing

    D Introducing a streamlined method to assist with service delivery and identification of deficits

    E Improving identification of deficits as well as skilled intervention in successive steps

    F Key principles on which the protocol is based with emphasis on successive steps toward higher-level goals

    G Author's work history as it relates to the case studies and development for The Protocol

II Foundational Information

    A Overview and child psychology basis of the development of The Protocol

    B Introduction to the point of interest concept, which is a high motivation factor when delivering services to our clients

    C Review of 'get on their level' and meeting a client where they are currently functioning along with their particular and independent interests

    D Answering the 'why' behind intervention

    E Reframing the 'why' question as it relates to our interventions and further our sharing of the information with parents and family members of the clients we serve

    F Discussed the association between cognitive milestones as outlined in the protocol and behaviors we see as educators and speech-language pathologists

    G Overview of language scaffolding and modeling procedures

H Review of interventions that are based on psychological factors
I Review of considerations related to non-English speakers during assessment and intervention planning

III Piaget's Stages

A Overview of what Piaget's stages encompass
B Review of Piaget and brief background provided
C Breakdown of the following four stages in detail: sensorimotor, pre-operational, concrete operational, formal operational
D Considerations that some children may never meet the later developing stages due to intellectual difficulties
E Consideration that while ages are provided, they are not always applicable or helpful due to a child's potential deficits
F Review of causes of deficits in any of the Piagetian stages
G Case study sample milestone score with intervention included
H Important collaborative considerations including special educators and referral for ABA (applied behavioral analysts) to assist with discrete trial training and academic and cognitive factors
I Preferred methods and procedures – in brief

IV Parten's Social Stages of Play

A Overview of what Parten's stages encompass
B Review of Parten and brief background provided
C Breakdown of the following stages in detail: unoccupied play, onlooker play, solitary play, cooperative play
D Considerations that some children may never meet the later developing stages due to intellectual difficulties or differences
E Consideration related to pragmatic deficits (concerns related to social skills), of which some areas of play need to be explicitly taught by the speech pathologist
F Review of causes of deficits in any of the Parten play stages
G Case study samples milestone score with intervention included
H Important collaborative considerations including special educators and referral for ABA (applied behavioral analysts)
I Preferred methods and procedures – in brief

V Cognitive Milestones

A Overview of what cognitive milestones encompass and the importance of identifying where a child lies
B Breakdown of the stages as they relate to receptive and expressive areas as well as basic functioning

C Considerations that the particular area of the protocol ceiling's out at basic cognitive skills which are reached at 5 years of age

D Review of causes of deficits that can impact a child's cognitive functioning

E Case study samples milestone score with intervention included

F Important collaborative considerations including special educators and psychological referrals for more detailed testing (tests which are commonly utilized in the United States)

G Preferred methods and procedures – in brief

VI Receptive Language Milestones

A Overview of what receptive milestones encompass and the importance of identifying where a child lies

B Breakdown of the stages as they relate to direction following and how this will present itself to a parent and educator

C Considerations that the particular area of the protocol ceiling's out at basic receptive language skills which are reached at 3–4 years of age, state that more advanced receptive language skills are covered in areas like Brown's morphemes and complexities chapter

D Review of causes of deficits that can impact a child's receptive language functioning

E Case study samples milestone score with intervention included

F Important collaborative considerations including audiologists (due to potential hearing concerns) and special educators

VII Expressive Language Milestones

A Overview of what expressive milestones encompass and the importance of identifying where a child lies

B Breakdown of the stages as there are many ways to 'express' oneself other than verbalizations – review of gestures and facial expressions

C Considerations that the particular area of the protocol ceiling's out at basic expressive language skills which are reached at 12–24 months of age, state that more advanced expressive language skills are covered in areas like Brown's morphemes and complexities chapter

D Review of causes of deficits that can impact a child's expressive language functioning

E Case study samples milestone score with intervention included

F Important collaborative considerations including audiologists (due to potential hearing concerns), special educators, and AAC experts (augmentative alternative communication)

VIII Motor Speech Progressions

    A Overview of what motor speech progressions encompass and the importance of identifying where a child lies

    B Breakdown of the stages as they relate to level of complexity

    C Review of causes of deficits that can impact a child's motor speech programming and coarticulation

    D Brief overview of childhood apraxia of speech, as it can relate to this and mention of adults speech sound production as well

    E Case study samples milestone scores and explicit examples with interventions included

    F Important collaborative considerations including physical and occupational therapy collaboration (due to gross and fine motor deficits in other areas)

    G Preferred methods and procedures – in brief

IX Speech Sounds and Phonological Norms

    A Overview of what speech sound errors encompass and the importance of identifying where a child lies

    B Overview of the stages as they relate to level of complexity

    C Review of causes of deficits that can impact a child's articulation

    D Common tests those in the United States are familiar with to probe further

    E Brief overview of differences across languages, as different languages have various speech sounds and ages of acquisition and mastery

    F Touch on relevance of speech sounds to the particular client who needs services (e.g. speech sounds in their name)

    G Case study samples milestone scores and explicit examples with interventions included

    H Important collaborative considerations including academic teachers and audiologists

    I Preferred methods and procedures – in brief

X Swallowing and Feeding Milestones

    A Overview of what swallowing and feeding milestones encompass and the importance of identifying where a child lies

    B Brief overview of dysphagia and concerns related to aspiration in comparison to sensory-based deficits that impact texture, taste, shape, color, etc.

    C Overview of the stages as they relate to the level of complexity and medical implications of deficits in this area

    D Review of causes of deficits that can impact a child's swallowing and feeding abilities

E Case study samples milestone scores and explicit examples with interventions included

F Important collaborative considerations including pediatrician referral, considerations for MBSS (modified barium swallow study), and occupational therapist and potential physical therapist referral

G Preferred methods and procedures – in brief

XI Social and Emotional Milestones

A Overview of what social and emotional milestones encompass and the importance of identifying where a child lies

B Overview of the stages as they relate to social interactions and attachment to others that are healthy

C Referral back to previously discussed milestones (e.g. Piaget's and cognitive milestones)

D Review of common deficit including children with autism spectrum disorder

E Review of causes of deficits that can impact social and emotional milestones

F Case study samples milestone scores and explicit examples with interventions included

G Important collaborative considerations including ABA therapy (applied behavioral analysts), sign language specialists, and specialized instructors

H Preferred methods and procedures – in brief

XII Social Communication Benchmarks

A Overview of what social communication benchmarks encompass and the importance of identifying where a child lies

B Overview of the stages as they relate to pragmatics (social skills)

C Reference to stages expanding to school age (12 years of age)

D Brief review of metalinguistic skills (higher level language skills), which will be delved into on the sequential charts

E Review of common deficit including children with autism spectrum disorder

F Review of causes of deficits that can impact pragmatic deficits

G Case study samples milestone scores and explicit examples with interventions included

H Important collaborative considerations including parents, peers, teachers, sports instructors and coaches, and occupational and physical therapists

I Preferred methods and procedures – in brief

XIII Brown's Stages of Morphological Development

A Overview of Roger Brown and his research which supports advancing complexity of language

B Overview of what syntactic and morphological areas encompass and the importance of identifying where a child lies

C Review of MLU (mean length of utterance) and golden rule as it relates to a child's age

D Reference to stages expanding to increasing linguistic complexities

E Review of common deficit including children who have specific language impairments and are learning English as a second language

F Case study samples milestone scores and explicit examples with interventions

G Important collaborative considerations including specialized instructors and collaboration with academic advisors (as it relates to literacy skills)

H Preferred methods and procedures – in brief

Appendix B
The Protocol Scoring Sheet

Name:
Date of Birth:
Date of Test:
Chronological Age:

Stage	Description	Goal of Stage	Age	Acquired? If So Which Portion (All, Some)
Sensorimotor stage	Learns through moving and exploring environment (object permanence, self-recognition, deferred imitation, and representational play) Emergency of symbolic function	Object permanence (requires ability to form mental representation – schema of object) – toward end of stage use one object to stand for another - Language begins because it's used to represent objects and feelings	Birth – 18/24 months	

(Continued)

(Continued)

Stage	Description	Goal of Stage	Age	Acquired? If So Which Portion (All, Some)
Preoperational stage	Internally represent world through language/ mental imagery; demonstration of animism	Symbolic thought	2–7 years	
Concrete operational stage	Logical thinking about concrete events; understand concept of conservation (certain properties remain the same); think more about how others think and feel	Logical thought	7–11 years	
Formal operational stage	Can deal with abstract ideas (e.g. fractions); follow an argument without specific examples; deal with hypothetical problems	Scientific reasoning	Adolescence to adults	

Mildred Parten (1932) Social Stages of Play

Stage of Development	Description	Age of Acquisition	Acquired (Y, N, Developing)
Solitary play	Play is solo; with their own ties. They don't typically get close to or interact with other children	Birth – 2 years	
Onlooker play	Child watching but not making attempt to join	Birth +	

(Continued)

(Continued)

Stage of Development	Description	Age of Acquisition	Acquired (Y, N, Developing)
Parallel play	Play is still solo but often next to (or parallel) to others	2.5–3.5 years	
Associative play	Begin to play with others by sharing toys (still may have their own play-line)	3–4.5 years	
Cooperative play	Children play in groups cooperatively to achieve common goal. Requires negotiation (where children can change roles/take turns and accept suggestions about play)	4–5.5 years	
Games with rules	Cooperative play that includes winners and losers. Children make the rules to these games (not like competitive sports). Demonstrate understanding of social rules in culture	6+ years	

Cognitive Milestones as reported by the CDC (of which 75% of the sampled population can do at the approximate age listed)

Milestone	Typical Age of Acquisition	Acquired (All, Some)
Watches caregiver as they move	2 months	
Looks at toy for several seconds	2 months	
Opens mouth for bottle if hungry	4 months	
Looks at own hands with interest	4 months	
Puts items in mouth to explore them	4 months	
Reaches to grab at desired toys	4 months	

(*Continued*)

(Continued)

Milestone	Typical Age of Acquisition	Acquired (All, Some)
Will demonstrate he's done with food by closing mouth	4 months	
Looks for toys/preferred items that are out of sight (object permanence)	9 months	
Bangs two items together	9 months	
Puts items in a container (e.g. block in a cup)	12 months	
Looks for items he sees you hide (e.g. stuffy under a blanket)	12 months	
Interacts with items the right way (demonstrates functional knowledge of items) (e.g. tries to talk on phone, will know to eat banana)	15 months	
Will stack at least two items (e.g. two blocks)	15 months	
Copies chores or routine activities (e.g. sweeping the floor, cleaning the dishes)	18 months	
Plays in toys in simple ways (e.g. pushing car)	18 months	
Can hold one item in one hand while simultaneously using the other hand to do something else (e.g. holding a cup and pouring with a teacup with the other hand)	2 years	
Attempts to use switches, knobs, zippers on toys	2 years	
Plays with more than one toy at a time (e.g. can take food out of play microwave and put it on a plate)	2 years	
Begins pretend play (e.g. feeding baby doll)	30 months	
Demonstrates simple problem-solving skills (e.g. stands on stool to reach counter)	30 months	

(*Continued*)

(Continued)

Milestone	Typical Age of Acquisition	Acquired (All, Some)
Follows two-step directions (e.g. get your shoes and bring them to the door)	30 months	
Knows at least one color (e.g. show me blue)	30 months	
Can draw a circle with direct model	3 years	
Avoids touching hot stove when given warning (safety awareness)	3 years	
Can label a number of colors	4 years	
Basic sequencing skills (can tell you what happens next in a familiar storybook)	4 years	
Draws a person with 3+ body parts	4 years	
Counts to 10	5 years	
Can label some colors when pointed to (from 1 to 5)	5 years	
Demonstrates understanding of time by using temporal words (e.g. yesterday, tomorrow, today)	5 years	
Can attend for 5–10 minutes on one task	5 years	
Writes some letters in their name	5 years	
Can name some letters when pointed to	5 years	

I. Receptive Language Milestones

Milestone	Age of Mastery	Acquired (Yes, No, Approaching/Scattered)
Startle or cry to unexpected noise	Birth	
Wake up to loud noises	Birth	
Stop moving upon hearing new and unfamiliar noises	Birth	
Turn head toward caregivers voice	3 months	

(*Continued*)

(Continued)

Milestone	Age of Mastery	Acquired (Yes, No, Approaching/Scattered)
Smile when hear parents voice	3 months	
Stop what they are doing and listen closely to a new noise	0–3 months	
Respond to comforting tone of voice (familiar or not)	0–3 months	
Respond to "no"	4–6 months	
Respond to different tones of voice	4–6 months	
Responds to noises other than talking (e.g. car driving by)	4–6 months	
Attends to toys and objects that make noise	4–6 months	
Enjoy music and rhythm	4–6 months	
Responds to their name (by turning and looking at the person calling them)	7–12 months	
Enjoys and attempts to participate in simple games (e.g. patty cake)	7–12 months	
Recognize the name of familiar objects (e.g. car, cookie, shoe)	7–12 months	
Imitates non-speech sounds (e.g. animal sounds "moo" "beep")	9–12 months	
Identifies pictures	12–15 months	
Displays object use (e.g. knows what to do with a cup, ball)	12–15 months	
Follows 1-step directions	21–24 months	
Points to pictures in a book once named	1–2 years	
Can point to a few body parts (e.g. nose, mouth, ear)	1–2 years	
Follows simple commands (e.g. "push the car")	1–2 years	
Understands simple questions (e.g. "where's the car?")	1–2 years	
Listens to simple stories	1–2 years	
Enjoys songs and rhymes	1–2 years	
Enjoys repetition of favored stories/songs and rhymes	1–2 years	
Identifies clothing items and their pictures	18–21 months	
Understands "come here" direction	18–21 months	
Uses two-word phrases	18–21 months	

(*Continued*)

(Continued)

Milestone	Age of Mastery	Acquired (Yes, No, Approaching/Scattered)
Understands 2-step directions (e.g. "get your shirt and put it in the hamper")	2–3 years	
Understands contrasting concepts (e.g. big/small, hot/cold)	2–3 years	
Recognized doorbell ringing or phone (demonstrated by pointing and showing excitement)	2–3 years	
Understands simple "who," "where," and "what" questions	2–3 years	
Can hear you and come when you call from another room (out of sight)	2–3 years	
Can answer simple 'wh' questions about stories	3–4 years	
Demonstrates understanding of the conversations going on at home, daycare, etc.	3–4 years	

I. Expressive Language Milestones

Milestone	Age of Mastery	Acquired? Yes, No, Some?
Make different sounds for pleasure or pain	0–3 months	
Smiles upon seeing caregiver	0–3 months	
Coo's or goo's or makes same sound when happy	0–3 months	
Produces different cries for different reasons (e.g. pain, hungry)	0–3 months	
Turns head to voices	3–6 months	
Babbles and laughs	3–6 months	
Produces /b, p, m/ consonants	3–6 months	
Gurgling or vocal play when entertained	4–6 months	
Begin babbling (begins with bilabials /p, b, w, m/)	4–6 months	
Uses sounds and gestures to indicate what they want	4–6 months	
Attends to pictures	6–9 months	
Attends to singing	6–9 months	
Responds to sounds of things he/she can't see	6–9 months	

(*Continued*)

(Continued)

Milestone	Age of Mastery	Acquired? Yes, No, Some?
More advanced babbling (new consonants and CV combinations with both long and short vowels)	7–12 months	
Uses speech or other sounds (other than crying) to get parents attention and communicate needs	7–12 months	
Imitates non-speech sounds (e.g. animal sounds "moo" "beep")	9–12 months	
First words or first word approximations! (e.g. "mama, night night")	7–12 months	
Shakes head "no"	12–15 months	
Names objects (e.g. ball, cup, milk)	12–15 months	
Labels 6 body parts	15–18 months	
Asks for "more"	15–18 months	
Verbalizes for various reasons (e.g. wants, needs, emotions)	18–21 months	
Uses 50–100 words	21–24 months	
Uses plurals	21–24 months	

Motor Speech Progressions

Complexity of Coarticulation	Acquired? Y/N, Emerging
Vowels	
CV's (animal sounds/ environmental noises)	
CVC's (simple words)	
Multisyllabic words	
1+ word utterances	
Sentence length	

Speech Sound Productions

Age of Mastery	Consonant Sounds	Acquired (Y/N)
2:0–2:11	/b, n, m, p, h, w, d/	
3:0–3:11	/g, k, f, t, ng, j/	
4:0–4:11	/v, dge(judge), s, ch, l, sh, z/	
5:0–5:11	/r, voiceless th(think), ge (television)/	
6:0–6:11	/voiced th(with)/	

Phonological Process	Description	Age of Elimination (Years)	Exhibited (Y/N)
Velar assimilation	Non-velars change to velars (due to their proximity to velars in the word) – e.g. /guck –duck/	3	
Nasal assimilation	Non-nasal sounds change to nasals (due to their proximity to nasal sounds in the word) – e.g. nunny – bunny	3	
Final consonant deletion	Deletion of the final consonant of a word – e.g. bu – bus	3	
Stopping	Fricative or affricate is replaced with a stopped sound – e.g. pun – fun	3–5 (depending on sounds)	
Fronting	Sounds made in back of mouth (velar) replaced with sounds produced in front of mouth – e.g. tar – car	4	
Deaffrication	Affricate replaced with fricative – e.g. ship – chip	4	
Cluster reduction	Consonant cluster is simplified with a single consonant – e.g. top – stop	4–5	
Weak syllable deletion	Unstressed/weak syllable in a word is deleted – e.g. nana – banana	4	
Gliding	Liquid sounds (/r/, /l/) replaced with glide (/w/ /j/) – e.g. wabbit– rabbit	6–7	

I. Swallowing and Feeding Milestones/Flowchart for Treatment

Age	Acquired Skills	Acquired (Y/N)
2–6 months	Hand on bottle during feeding	
4–6 months	Maintains semi-flexed posture	
6 months	Sitting with support	
4–6 months	Semi-flexed posture during feeding	
6–9 months (transitory feeding)	Sitting independently for time	
6–9 months	Self-oral stimulation (mouthing hands and toys)	

(Continued)

(Continued)

Age	Acquired Skills	Acquired (Y/N)
	Spoon feeding (thin, smooth puree)	
	Suckle pattern (initially suck, swallow)	
	Both hands hold bottle	
	Pincer grasp (crawling on all fours)	
	Finger feeding (introduced)	
	Vertical munching (dissolvable solids)	
	Prefers parents to feed	
9–12 months (first steps, cruising along furniture)	Cup drinking	
	Eats lumpy mashed food	
	Finger feeding (dissolvable solids)	
	Rotary chew action	
	Assisting with spoon feeding	
12–18 months (refined gross and fine motor skills)	Self-feeding (grasps spoon with whole hand)	
	Holds cup with both hands	
	Drinking with 4–5 consecutive swallows	
	Holding and tipping bottle	
> 18–24 months	Swallowing with lip closure	
	Self-feeding predominates	
	Chewing varied range of food textures	
	Up and down tongue movements	
	More precise chew pattern	
24–36 months	Circulatory jaw rotations	
	Chewing with lip closure	
	Holds cup with one hand	
	Open cup drinking without spillage	
	Uses fingers to fill spoon	
	Eats wide range of solids	
	Independent feeding – using fork	

Social-Emotional Developmental Milestones

Social interaction	Typical age of acquisition	Mastered y/n/developing
Smile at people	2 months	
Can briefly calm selves (sucking on hands)	2 months	
Try to look at parents	2 months	
Smile spontaneously at people	4 months	
Enjoying playing with others (can cry when stops)	4 months	
Copy some movements and facial expressions (e.g. frowning)	4 months	
Know familiar faces (and strangers)	6 months	
Respond to others emotions		
Like to look at self in mirror	6 months	
Fear of strangers	9 months	
Cry when parents leave	1 year	
Verbalize for attention (repeat words or sounds)	1 year	
Play interactive games (e.g. 'pat a cake')	1 year	

Social Communication "Benchmarks" (ASHA)

Birth–12 months

Action	Acquired
Prefers looking at human face and eyes	
Prefers human voices	
Looks for source of sound	
Differentiates between tones of voice (angry/friendly)	
Smiles back at caregiver	
Follows caregivers gaze	
Participates in preverbal vocal turn-taking	
Vocalizes to gain attention	
Demonstrates joint attention skills (sharing attention	

(*Continued*)

(Continued)

Uses gestures to make requests and
 direct attention
Plays simple interactive games
 (peekaboo)
Seeks comfort from caregiver
Expresses feelings
Develops object permanence
Discriminates facial expressions
Fear of strangers
Relational memory develops (faces/
 voices)
Changes behavior to achieve goal
Imitates gestures/oral movements

12–18 months

Range of communicative intentions
 (requests, comments)
Brings objects to show caregivers
Requests via pointing and vocalizing
Gains attention by vocalizing
Practices vocal inflection
Says "bye" and other ritualized
 greetings
Protests by shaking head and
 saying "no"
Uses gestures with verbal language
Demonstrates awareness of the social
 value of speech
Responds to others' speech by giving
 eye contact
Demonstrates sympathy, empathy, and
 sharing nonverbally
Shows joy, fear, and anger
Increase in autonomy
Resists control
Co-regulates interactions

18–24 months

Uses single words to express intention
Single and paired words to command,
 indicate possession, and gain
 attention
Uses I, me, you, my, and mine
Participates in verbal turn taking
 (limited turns)

(*Continued*)

(Continued)

Demonstrates simple topic control
Interrupts at syntactic junctures or in
  response to prosodic cues
Demonstrates secure and insecure
  attachment pattern
Exhibits emotion and behavioral
  regulation
Demonstrates increase in autonomy
Develops emerging implicit perceptual
  access reasoning
Shows daily routine schemes in play

24–36 months

Engages in short dialogues

Verbally introduces and changes topic
Expresses emotion
Begins to use language in
  imaginative way
Relates own experiences
Begins to include descriptive details to
  enhance listeners understanding
Uses attention-getting words
Clarifies and asks for clarification
Uses politeness terms or markers
Begins to demonstrate adaptation of
  speech to different audience/listeners
Can deceive and detect deception
Understands that others may feel
  differently than themselves
Follows rules
Shoes common but not daily schemes
  in play (e.g. doctor, shopping)
Uses embedded requests

3–4 years

Engages in longer dialogues
Anticipates next turn at talking
Terminates conversation; appropriately
  role-plays
Uses filers (e.g. "yeah" "okay") to
  acknowledge partners message
Begins code-switching and using
  simpler language when talking to
  very young children

(*Continued*)

(Continued)

Uses elliptical responses (e.g. "mommy
  went home, I didn't"
Requests permission
Begins using language for fantasies,
  jokes, and teasing
Makes conversational repairs when not
  understood and correct others
Infers information from a story and
  infers indirect meanings
Uses primitive narratives – events
  follow from central core
Uses inferences in stories

4–5 years

Uses indirect requests; correctly uses
  deictic terms (e.g. this, that, there,
  here)
Uses twice as many effective utterances
  as 3-year-olds to discuss emotions
  and feelings
Uses narrative development
  characterized by unfocused
  chains – stories have a sequence of
  events but no central character or
  theme
Develops basic understanding of theory
  of mind, including judgment that
  another person may have a belief
  that differs from the truth
Shifts topics rapidly
Shows fantasy schemes in play
Understands that beliefs can result in
  predictable emotions
Understands that someone may feel
  the same way when experiencing
  a similar event
Uses comissives/promises

School-age Years (6–12 years)

Demonstrates increased understanding
  of theory of mind (predicting what
  one person is thinking about what
  another person is thinking or feeling;
  understands strategies to hide deceit,
  recognizes sarcasm)

(*Continued*)

(Continued)

Provides assistance and demonstrates
  altruism
Uses narrative development
  characterized by causally sequenced
  events using "story grammar"
Demonstrates improved conversational
  skills (e.g. topic maintenance, repair,
  increased number of turns)
Extends topic of conversation
Demonstrates refined social
  conventions
Demonstrates metapragmatic
  skills – child is able to think about
  social and conversational rules
Uses language for varied functions,
  including persuading and advancing
  one's opinion
Understands that people can feel
  multiple emotions at the same time
Practices increased self-regulation
Uses indirect requests
Uses inferential language
Uses ambiguous language (figurative)
Uses sarcasm
Uses double meanings (puns)

The Protocol Analysis

Piaget's Stages

Level of mastery
Zone of intervention
Age expectancy

Social Stages of Play

Level of mastery
Zone of intervention
Age expectancy

Cognitive

Level of mastery
Zone of intervention
Age expectancy

(Continued)

Receptive Language

Level of mastery
Zone of intervention
Age expectancy

Expressive Language

Level of mastery
Zone of intervention
Age expectancy

Motor Speech Progressions

Level of mastery
Zone of intervention
Age expectancy

Speech Sounds

Level of mastery
Zone of intervention
Age expectancy

Swallowing and Feeding

Level of mastery
Zone of intervention
Age expectancy

Social and Pragmatic

Level of mastery
Zone of intervention
Age expectancy

Brown's Stages

Level of mastery
Zone of intervention
Age expectancy

Social Communication

Level of mastery
Zone of intervention
Age expectancy

Index